THE INVISION GUIDE TO
A HEALTHY HEART

THE INVISION GUIDE TO

A HEALTHY HEART

ALEXANDER TSIARAS

Collins
An Imprint of HarperCollinsPublishers

HarperCollins books may be purchased for educational, business, or sales promotional use. For information, please write: Special Markets Department, HarperCollins Publishers, 10 East 53rd Street, New York, NY 10022.

FIRST EDITION

Designed by Cindy Goldstein, Eric Baker Design Associates

Library of Congress Cataloging-in-Publication Data
has been applied for.

ISBN-10   0-06-085593-2
ISBN-13   978-0-06-085593-2

05 06 07 08   09 / RRD   10 9 8 7 6 5 4 3 2

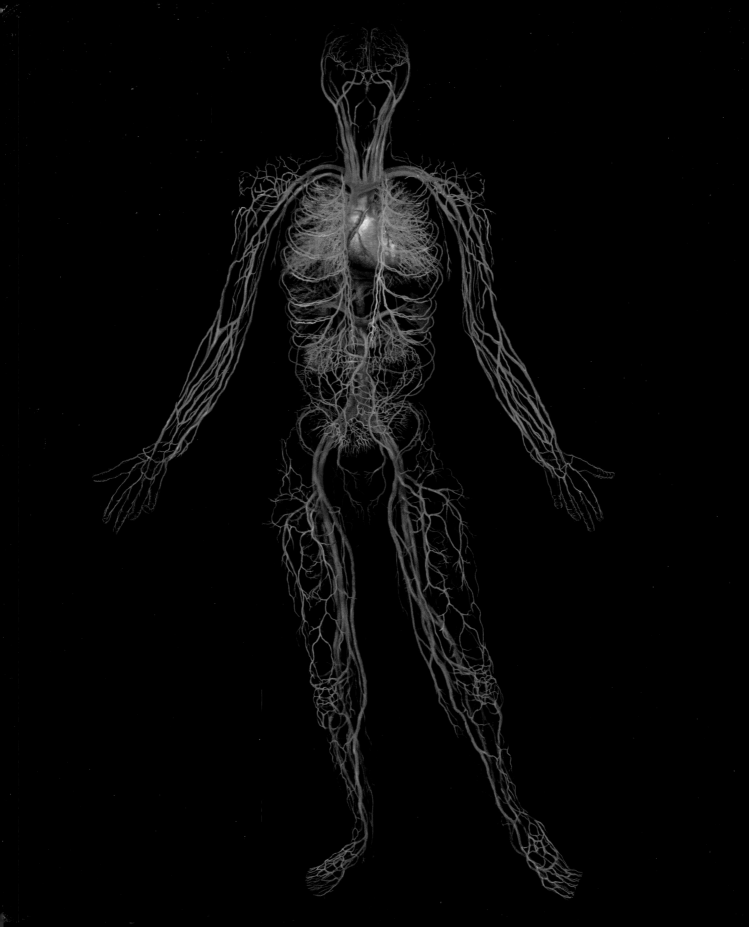

There is a great educational need in this country, one that hasn't been sufficiently fulfilled by the government, healthcare industry, or media. Public health education is currently not achieving its goals. Millions of people with chronic illnesses have no idea how and why their bodies are failing them; millions more are endangering their health through risk behaviors that can be modified. This book is the first in the InVision Guide series, a series that will visualize abnormalities of the human condition in a uniquely engaging format. As our first partner in the InVision Guide series, Novartis Pharmaceuticals Corporation is acknowledging its commitment to public health and wellness. We dedicate this book to Novartis and applaud them for having the vision to underwrite the research and development that has made this imagery available. Now, everyone—individuals, families, those at-risk—has access to and can be inspired by these high-end medical images that are coupled with clear explanations of the science of cardiovascular health. By encouraging the reader to both marvel at the beauty and complexity of his/her body while learning critical facts about cardiovascular health, this book represents a fresh approach to jump-starting a public awareness of treatments and preventative solutions.

—ALEXANDER TSIARAS

ACKNOWLEDGMENTS

Attila Ambrus, Creative Director/
Director of Scientific Visualization:
For his leadership, unique creative and technical skill, and numerous late hours in front of a keyboard.

Ann Canapary, Project Manager/Visualization Expert:
For her organizational skills, medical knowledge, artistic supervision, and dedication in the face of all the complexities that were thrown at her during this project.

Jeremy Mack, Associate Creative Director,
Department of Scientific Visualization:
For his originality and artistic supervision.

Poy Yee, Senior Designer:
For his creativity and design contributions.

I want to thank Shirley Chan, Ph.D., for her quick wit, true appreciation of the micromechanics of the human body, and her facile use of the English language.
Shirley is currently the Director of Educational Development and Interactive Media at Anatomical Travelogue Inc. She obtained her doctorate in molecular biology and genetics from the University of Toronto in Canada. Shirley ran the multimedia department at the Dolan DNA Learning Center at Cold Spring Harbor Laboratory and has written extensively on DNA, genetics, and cancer.

Jacquelyn Sun, Designer and Medical Visualization Specialist:
For her countless hours and problem-solving abilities.

Betty Lee, Jean-Claude Michel, Matt Wimsatt, and Jin Yoon, Medical Visualization Specialists:
For their artistry, long hours, creativity, and justified pride in their work.

Photographers: Eric Alba and Fabio Dozzini

Anatomical Travelogue Inc. staff:
Justine Angelis, Laszlo Balogh, Asena Basak, Nilufer Candar, Sharon Ching, Joshua Cohen, Stewart Deitch, Lloyd Fales, Lachlan Inglis, Ezra Kortz, Mark Mallari, Ildiko McGivney, Karina Metcalf, Gloria Situ, Casey Steffen and Attila Zalanyi

Models:
Vijay Amritraj, Stewart Deitch, Jill Gregory, Robert Henry, Chloe Lin, Vivian Matalon-Taub, Suzannah Matalon, Timea Resan, Judy Shane, Gloria Situ, Eden Taub, Kyla Taub, Gavin Whelan, Kate Wimsatt

On Camera:
Ryan Bendixen, Isobel Cargill, John Castaldo, M.D., Peter Fail, M.D., William Fitz-Gibbon, James Goodreau, M.D., Edna Lucas, John Lucas, Mehmet C. Oz, M.D., Donald J. Poskitt

Researchers:
Elizabeth Boskey and Sharon Ching

Contributing writers:
Elizabeth Bogner, Elizabeth Boskey, and Kathy Silberger

Eric Baker Design:
With a special thanks to Eric Baker and Cindy Goldstein for their continued originality and professionalism.

Novartis Pharmaceuticals Corporation for their scientific underwriting:
Special thanks to Anna Frable and Len Brandt at Novartis Pharmaceuticals Corporation for their constant support, efficiency, and belief in the best values of our effort to educate and inform.

Philips Electronics North America Corporation for medical imaging:
Special thanks to Terry Fassburg and Karin Daly for their support and access to their extraordinary data.

Toni Sciarra at Collins:
For her contributions that have elevated the quality of this book several notches.

Bob Levine, Levine Plotkin & Menin, LLP:
For his belief in our work and vision.

Carrie Liaskos and Charlotte Noble at Chandler Chicco Agency

Adrianne Noe, Director of the National Museum of Health and Medicine of the AFIP

National Institutes of Health

National Library of Medicine and the Visible Human project

National Museum of Health and Medicine of the AFIP

Scientific Visualization Software developed in collaboration with Volume Graphics, GmbH, Germany (http://www.volumegraphics.com)

To the scientific advisory board, who were instrumental in the accuracy and direction of the science and imagery that has pushed the limits of Anatomical Travelogue's technology. We thank them:

Gregory W. Albers, M.D., Professor of Neurology and Neurological Sciences, Stanford University Medical Center, Director, Stanford Stroke Center

Jay N. Cohn, M.D., Professor of Medicine, University of Minnesota Medical School

Kenneth A. Jamerson, M.D., Professor of Medicine, Division of CV Medicine, University of Michigan Healthcare System, Medical Director, Program for Multi-Cultural Health

Mehmet C. Oz, M.D., Professor and Vice-Chairman of Surgery and Director of the Heart Institute, New York Presbyterian, Columbia University

Biff F. Palmer, M.D., Professor of Internal Medicine, University of Texas Southwestern Medical School

James M. Rippe, M.D. Founder/Director, Rippe Lifestyle Institute, Shrewsbury, MA, Associate Professor of Medicine (Cardiology), Tufts University School of Medicine, Boston, MA

All stock imagery is from the Science Source division of Photo Researchers Inc., http://www.sciencesource.com.

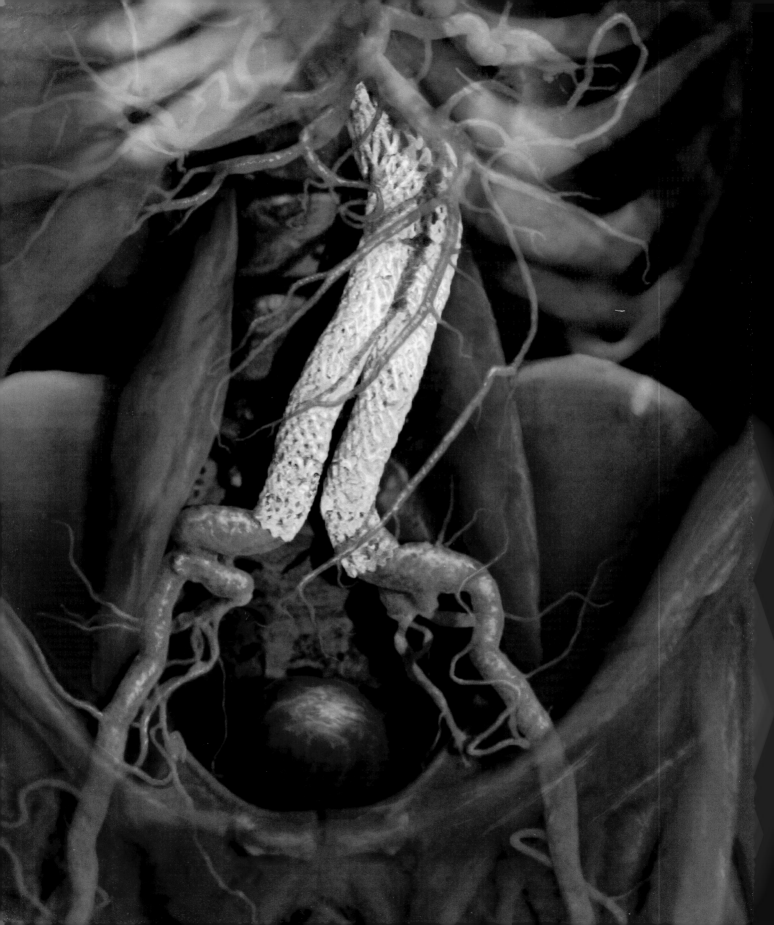

FOREWORD

Frequently artistic developments predate major advances in science and even create the fertile environment for their occurrence. For example, Impressionism surfaced in France in the 1870s and only three decades later did Einstein and other physicists propose that light energy was made of particles. Occasionally, science predates art by bringing new technologies into the public arena.

Alexander Tsiaras and his extraordinary staff of artists and scientists at Anatomical Travelogue have produced a remarkable creation. With this wonderful book, we witness the confluence of paradigms as the worlds of art and science are brought together and both advance in unison.

The past years have seen an explosion in our understanding and treatment of cardiovascular disease. We no longer are restricted to an understanding of the human body based on autopsy. Instead, innovative imaging techniques ranging from coronary angiography to state-of-the-art ultrafast computed tomography scans show us the inner workings of the living heart. We learn the importance of the inflamed plaque whose rupture causes so much havoc, and appreciate the impact of lifestyle changes on these processes. The ravages of subtle human conditions like hypertension and diabetes can be exposed as we empower humans to control their health destiny. After all, one cannot have a wealthy society without a healthy society.

In this age of information, people are becoming more involved in their healthcare decisions and proactive in making informed life-altering decisions for their loved ones. However, many face the confusing reality of information—and misinformation—overload.

Millions of pages of text and poetry have been written about the heart, but the book you are holding in your hands is completely unique. The visuals represent the results of imaging technology so sophisticated as to be a decade ahead of availability even to medical professionals. A picture is worth a thousand words, and this book will show you stunning visuals of the amazing organ called the heart, and the intricate system it powers—in robust health, in trouble, and in treatment. Alexander Tsiaras and his group translate complex data—particularly medical images—and shape them into beautiful, approachable, and easy-to-understand visual narratives. The information used to create the images are actual human scans from MRIs, CTs, and ultrasounds—highly sophisticated diagnostic equipment. The scans start out as flat two-dimensional slices that are then digitized and reassembled to produce the three-dimensional images you see. Medical professionals are trained to interpret medical information from the two-dimensional perspective, but images like these, which have depth and context, make the information so much more immediate and intuitive. Not only can such images assist doctors in making diagnoses more easily and accurately, but they also make it much easier to share this intuitive data with colleagues, patients, and patients' families. This imaging process is truly revolutionary: in addition to being useful for diagnostic and educational purposes, the images are just plain beautiful.

In the chapters that follow, you will see the heart and cardiovascular system telling a striking visual story: there is a continuum of heart and cardiovascular development, from the very first heartbeat to the heart attack damage caused by a blocked artery. When the cardiovascular system is compromised, it's not just the heart that suffers. Through highly detailed images of the brain, kidneys, and other organs, you'll gain a vivid sense of how the body works, and how its intricately integrated systems support total well-being.

These images, accompanied by accessible explanations, case examples, and effective strategies for achieving cardiovascular health, offer a beautiful vision of the body. To have this wondrous body and fully participate in life is a joy, a wonder, an honor. To attain and maintain our health is a sacred charge each of us carries throughout our life.

I am delighted to have contributed to the creation of this project and hope you enjoy the results as much as we enjoy offering these glimpses of reality to you.
To your health,

Mehmet C. Oz, M.D.,
Professor and Vice Chairman,
Department of Surgery
New York Presbyterian-Columbia University

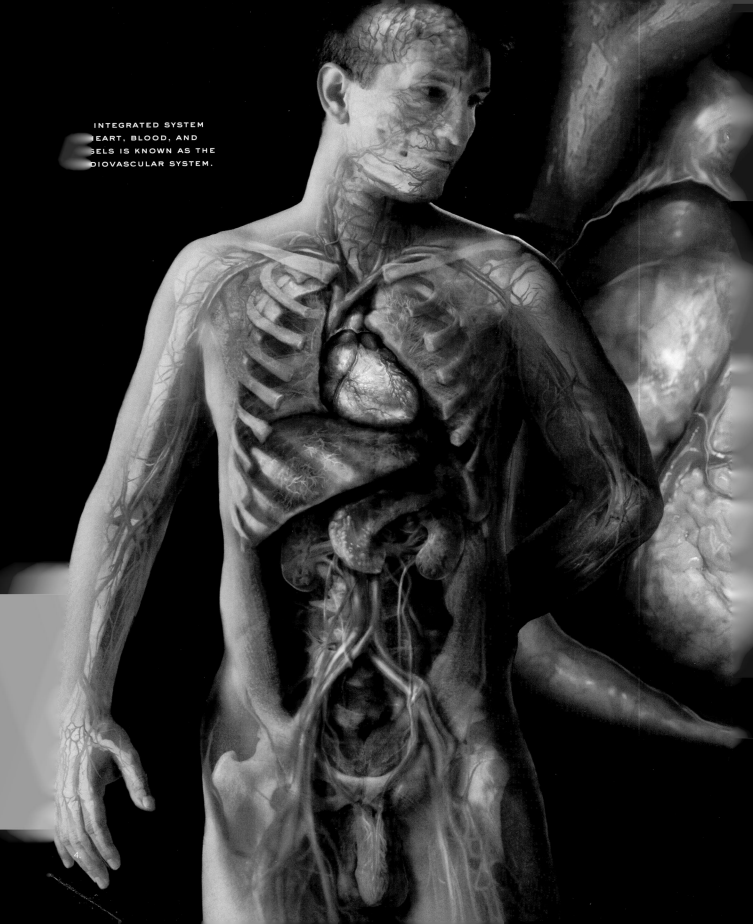

THE INTEGRATED SYSTEM
OF HEART, BLOOD, AND
VESSELS IS KNOWN AS THE
CARDIOVASCULAR SYSTEM.

4

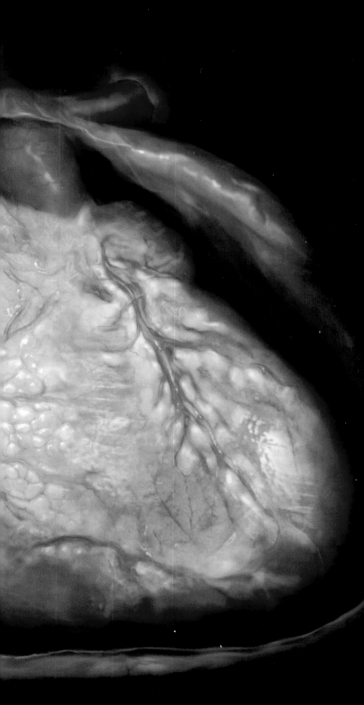

THE HEART IS CUSHIONED
WITHIN THE CHEST BY ITS OWN
LUBRICATED PROTECTIVE SAC

and the beat goes on:
developing a heart
and vascular system

The rosy pink of a newborn baby, the pulse at the base of your neck, the blush of pleasure or shame, the pins and needles in your fingers when you come in from the cold: these are all examples of a working cardiovascular system.

In the average adult, the heart beats 72 times a minute, 100,000 times a day, 3,500,000 times a year. Each heartbeat circulates blood through a huge network of vessels: arteries, veins, and capillaries. If the vessels in your body were stretched end to end, they would extend for 60,000 miles—enough to circle the globe two-and-a-half times. Yet, in the time it takes you to finish reading this page, all of the blood in your body will have circled through the system. During an average lifetime, the heart will pump about one million barrels of blood—enough to fill four supertankers.

The integrated system of heart, blood, and vessels is known as the cardiovascular system. It is our body's internal supply line and carries nutrients and information to all the different parts of the body. It is also our body's disposal network, collecting cellular waste products for elimination. Without an appropriately working cardiovascular system, we cannot regulate our body temperature, move, or even think.

This book uses real human data to take you on a tour of the cardiovascular system. You will see the incredible inner workings of your body from the very first heartbeat (pulse). You will also see some of the cardiovascular problems that you may encounter throughout your life, and learn how these are treated

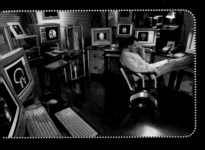

Alexander Tsiaras has spent more than 25 years developing techniques to visualize the human body. Using a special camera and data from different types of medical scans, he has been able to produce never-before-seen images of the developing embryo. Mr. Tsiaras: "In the first four weeks of embryonic development, there is an exponential growth of cells. All of this growth is coordinated so that the right cells end up in the right places doing the right things."

VOLUME RENDERING SOFTWARE CAN BE USED TO:

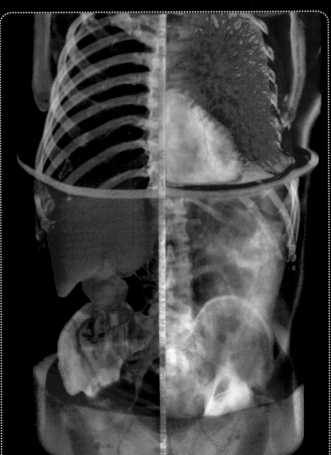

ISOLATE COMPLETE
BODY SYSTEMS
SUCH AS BONE.

EXAMINE 3D DETAILS
OF ANATOMICAL
STRUCTURES SUCH AS
BRONCHIOLES AND
CORONARY ARTERIES.

ISOLATE SOFT
TISSUE THAT
MAKE UP ORGANS
SUCH AS THE
LIVER AND KIDNEY.

SEE THROUGH THE
BODY USING A 3D
X-RAY TECHNIQUE.

THREE ISOLATED SLICES
FROM THE 300 THAT MAKE
UP THE HEART VOLUME.

FRONT OF THE HEART
REPRESENTING SEVERAL
DIFFERENT RENDERING
TECHNIQUES.

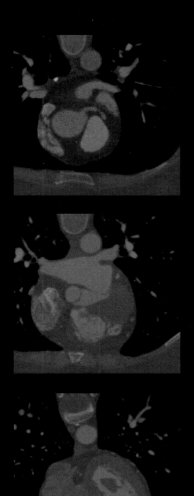

A

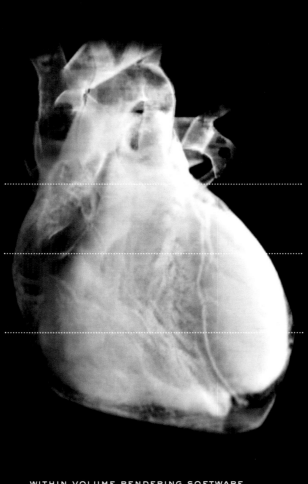

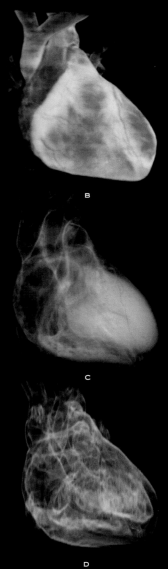

B

C

D

WITHIN VOLUME RENDERING SOFTWARE,
SLICES OF MAGNETIC RESONANCE IMAGERY
(MRI), AND COMPUTER TOMOGRAPHY (CT)
SCANS CAN BE COMPILED TO PRODUCE A
THREE-DIMENSIONAL (3D) MODEL OF AN
ORGAN SUCH AS A HEART. MODELS CAN BE
VIEWED AS (A) INDIVIDUAL SLICES, (B)
ENHANCED COLOR, (C) GRAY-SCALE VOLUME,
AND (D) 3D TRANSPARENCY.

4-WEEK-OLD EMBRYO

9-WEEK-OLD FETUS

5-MONTH-OLD FETUS

Contained entirely within the nurturing space of the womb, the developing embryo cannot eat or breathe, and therefore must obtain all nutrients from other sources. For the first nine weeks, the early embryo depends on the yolk sac for nourishment. Inside the yolk sac, tiny structures called blood islands form. These will become the first blood vessels. As pregnancy continues, these important external structures develop into the embryo's link to the mother's system—the umbilical cord and the supporting network known as the placenta. Until birth the fetus is completely dependent on the mother for nutrients and waste disposal through the umbilical cord and the placenta.

UMBILICAL CORD

PLACENTA

THE FETUS IS COMPLETELY
DEPENDENT ON THE MOTHER
FOR NUTRIENTS AND
WASTE DISPOSAL THROUGH
THE UMBILICAL CORD AND
THE PLACENTA.

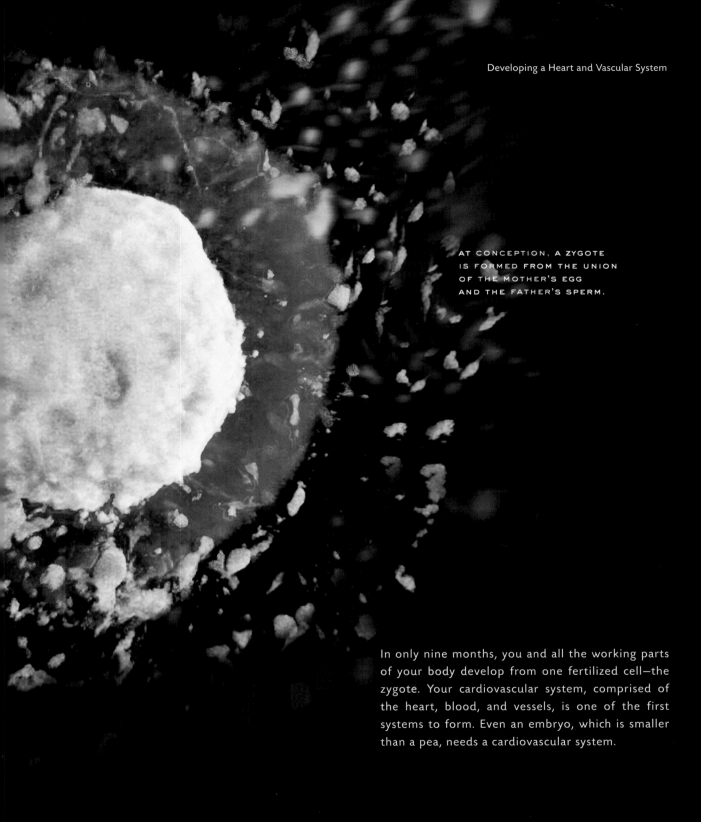

AT CONCEPTION, A ZYGOTE
IS FORMED FROM THE UNION
OF THE MOTHER'S EGG
AND THE FATHER'S SPERM.

In only nine months, you and all the working parts of your body develop from one fertilized cell—the zygote. Your cardiovascular system, comprised of the heart, blood, and vessels, is one of the first systems to form. Even an embryo, which is smaller than a pea, needs a cardiovascular system.

5-WEEK-OLD EMBRYO

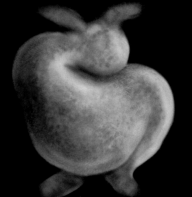

HEART ···

A

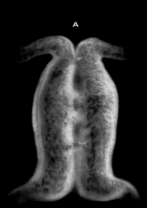

By the 25th day of gestation, a heart is already pumping and circulating blood through a network of vessels. These initial heartbeats come from a very different organ than the one seen in an adult. This early heart is really only a simple tube twisted back on itself (A) because there is not enough room to grow. By the 5th week, the twisted tube fuses and becomes a two-chambered heart with one atrium and one ventricle (B). By the 6th week, a vertical wall—known as the septum—grows up the middle of the two chambers (C, D), dividing them to form the four-chambered heart that will continue into adulthood (E).

B

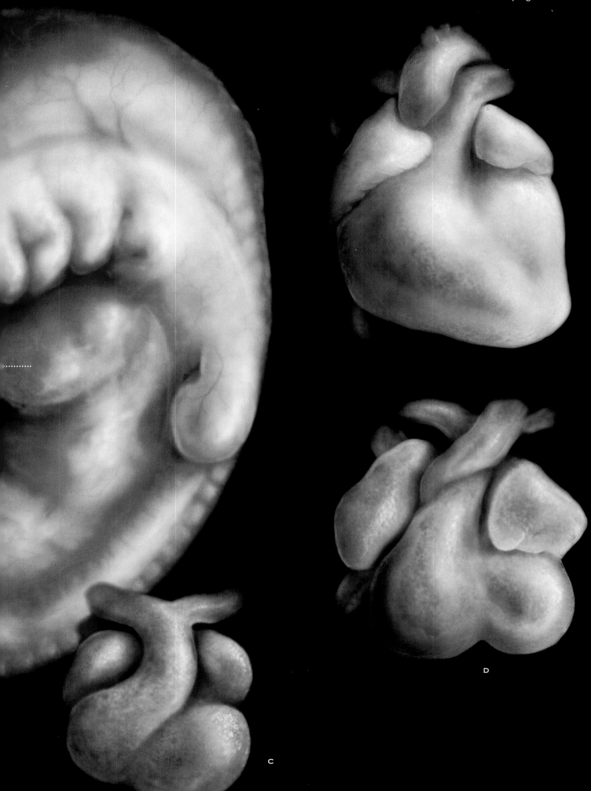

E

D

C

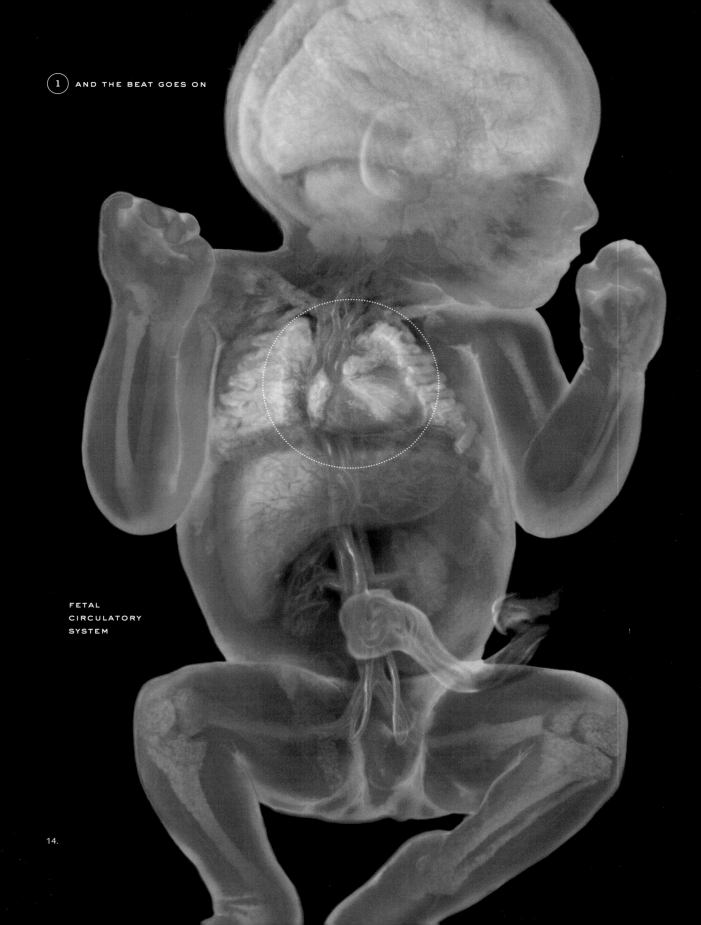

FETAL
CIRCULATORY
SYSTEM

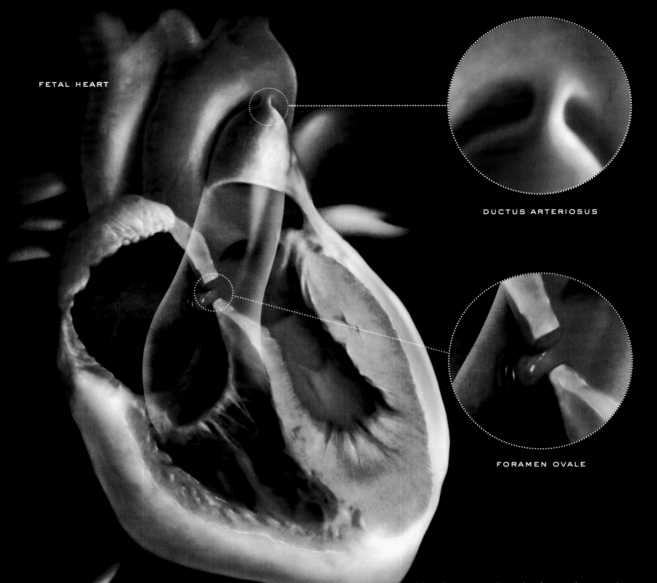

FETAL HEART

DUCTUS ARTERIOSUS

FORAMEN OVALE

After birth, the right and left sides of your heart do different things. The right side of the heart collects blood and pumps it into the lungs so that the blood can pick up oxygen (oxygenation) and dispose of carbon dioxide. The oxygenated blood passes through the lung to the left side of the heart. This is known as pulmonary circulation. The left side of the heart pumps the oxygenated blood out to the rest of the body. The body tissues extract oxygen and nutrients and deposit waste, including carbon dioxide, into the blood. This deoxygenated blood is then returned to the right heart. This is known as systemic circulation.

Circulation operates differently in the fetus. While a fetus is developing in the womb, the lungs never expand and never collect or contain any air.

Oxygenated blood comes directly from the mother through the placenta and umbilical cord. In addition, the path of blood through the fetal heart is different from that of an adult. In the fetus, much of the blood that enters the right side of the heart flows directly into the left side of the heart through an opening called the *foramen ovale* and back out into the body. The remaining blood that flows into the major vessel to the lungs—the pulmonary artery—is redirected away from the non-functioning lungs. It moves directly from the pulmonary artery through a pathway called the *ductus arteriosus* into the major vessel to the rest of the body—the aorta. Although the vessels are in place and the four-chambered heart works, until birth, blood circulating through the fetus bypasses the pulmonary circulation.

15.

Birth is miraculous in more ways than one.
Alexander Tsiaras: "At the moment of birth, you're separating yourself from your mobile heart/lung/immunology machine and within seconds you have to activate your own systems: breathe on your own, process your own foods, and fight your own germ battles. And because of how you live and the aging process, never again will your cardiovascular system be as pristine as the day you're born. This is the gold standard of cardiovascular health."

THE INFANT WILL TAKE HIS/HER FIRST BREATH SECONDS AFTER BIRTH.

The lungs of an unborn child are one of the last organs to complete development. This is, in part, due to the fact that the fetal lungs are not needed during pregnancy. The fetus exists in a fluid-filled womb and receives oxygenated blood from the mother. However, at birth, as soon as that first breath of air rushes into a baby's lungs, there is a drastic increase in the amount of blood flowing through the lungs. In the fetus, blood flows directly into the left side of the fetal heart. At birth, after the baby takes the first breath, all the blood that is pumped from the right side of the heart now must pass through the lungs to be oxygenated. After the first breath, the *foramen ovale* (the opening between the right and left sides of the heart) seals up and the right ventricle pumps the blood through the pulmonary artery into the lungs. The *ductus arteriosus* also closes, so that when the oxygenated blood returns to the left

16.

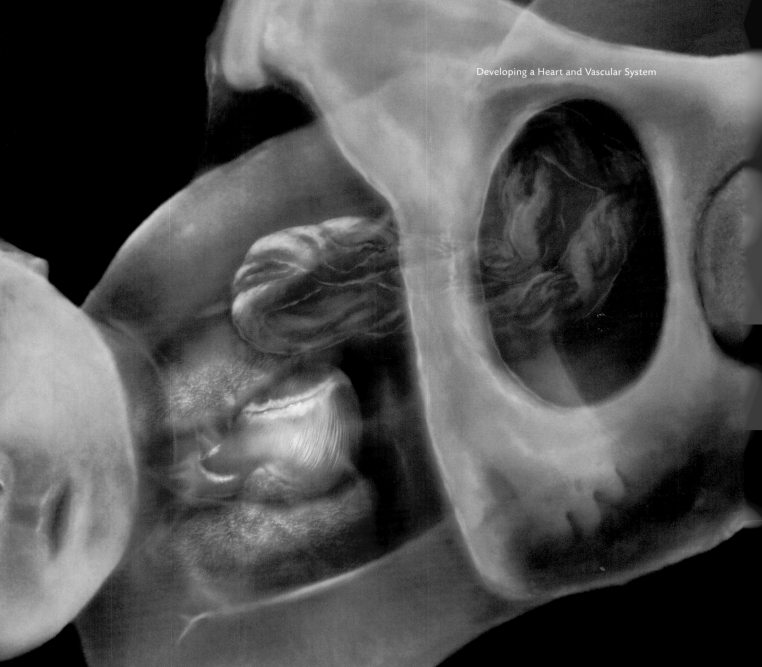

side of the heart from the lungs, the left ventricle pumps the blood through the aorta out to the rest of the body.

Deoxygenated blood flows into the right atrium, past the sealed *foramen ovale*, and into the right ventricle, where it is sent on its path for oxygenation. It makes its way through the pulmonary artery, and goes straight past the closed-off *ductus arteriosus* to pick up oxygen from the lungs. The oxygen-rich, red

blood then returns to the left atrium of the heart through the pulmonary vein, which shoots it into the left ventricle to be pumped through the aorta and out to the rest of the body. The blood goes out through the arteries, moves into the capillaries, and returns to the heart through the venules and veins. This is the circulatory path that blood will travel throughout one's lifetime.

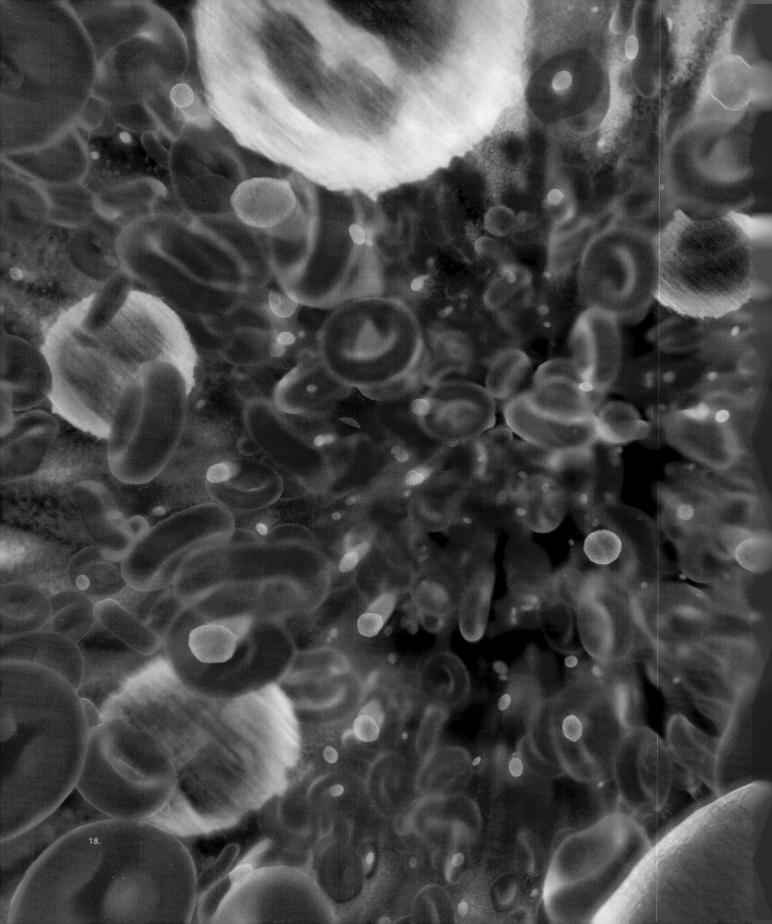

18.

2

**how things work:
the living pump and pipes**

The main job of your cardiovascular system is transport. Your heart pumps blood through the vessels to all parts of your body, delivering nutrients and taking away wastes. To do this efficiently, your cardiovascular system actually consists of two separate circulatory networks—pulmonary and systemic—working in tandem. The right side of your heart controls the pulmonary circulation while the left controls the systemic circulation. With these circulation networks, blood can travel through your entire body in about thirty seconds.

In general, no matter what happens to the rest of your body, important organs like your heart, brain, and kidneys attempt to maintain a constant supply of blood: 15 to 20% goes to the brain and the central nervous system; 5% supplies the heart; and 22% goes to the kidneys. The function of these organs is crucial. In the event of blood loss, circulation is decreased to other parts of the body first to minimize damage to these vital organs.

One of the most amazing things about the cardiovascular system is its ability to monitor the body and work differently in different situations. Whether you are exercising, standing on your head, or being exposed to the cold, your cardiovascular system is constantly monitoring itself and getting information about the needs of the body, which it uses to make necessary changes. For example, during exercise or high-stress situations, your breathing and heart rate increase. Your heart can pump twice as fast and circulate four times as much blood through your body. Your blood vessels can dilate and contract, diverting more blood flow to your muscles and less to your stomach. This balancing of your body's needs with the blood supply is controlled by both local tissue signals and information received from the brain.

YOUR CARDIOVASCULAR SYSTEM PUMPS BLOOD THROUGH YOUR BODY TO DELIVER NUTRIENTS, TAKE AWAY WASTES, FIGHT OFF ILLNESSES, AND HEAL INJURIES.

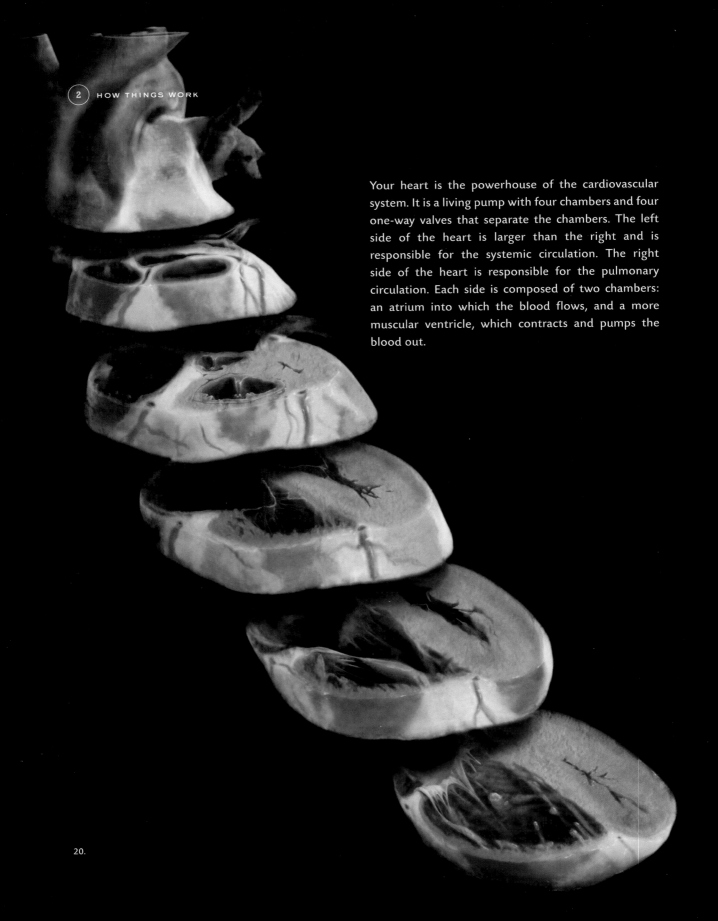

Your heart is the powerhouse of the cardiovascular system. It is a living pump with four chambers and four one-way valves that separate the chambers. The left side of the heart is larger than the right and is responsible for the systemic circulation. The right side of the heart is responsible for the pulmonary circulation. Each side is composed of two chambers: an atrium into which the blood flows, and a more muscular ventricle, which contracts and pumps the blood out.

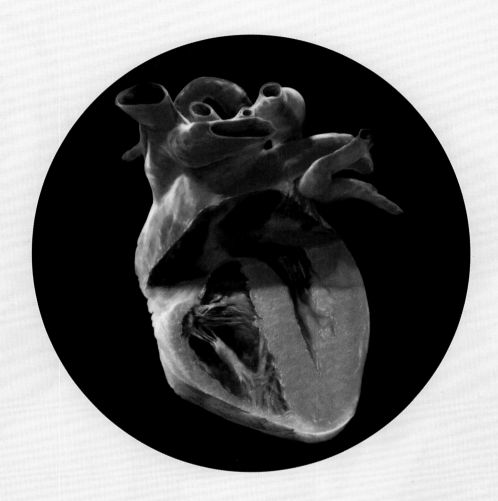

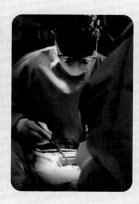

Mehmet Oz, M.D., is one of the top cardiac surgeons in the country. In his work at New York Presbyterian-Columbia University Hospital in New York City, he operates on more than 350 patients a year using the most advanced surgical techniques available. From robotic surgery to a wraparound stocking that prevents the heart from enlarging due to damage, Dr. Oz works on the leading edge of cardiovascular technology.

Dr. Oz has a very visual and visceral understanding of heart function. "Most folks think that the heart empties blood the way a balloon evacuates air. Absolutely wrong. The way the heart empties blood is the way you would wring water from a towel. You twist the blood out with your heart. And when you have heart damage, when the heart gets enlarged, one of the things that we lose is the efficiency of that twisting action. Instead of being able to twist effectively, one side doesn't help. Try twisting the water out of a towel with only one hand doing the twisting. It's a lot more difficult."

CLOSED   OPEN

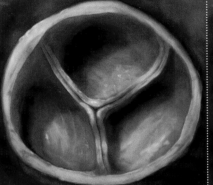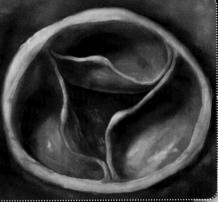

PULMONARY AND AORTIC VALVES

CLOSED   OPEN

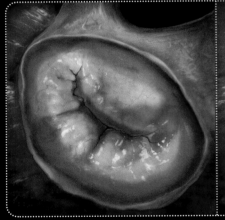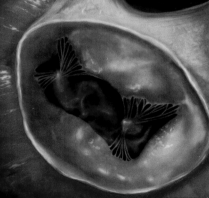

MITRAL VALVE

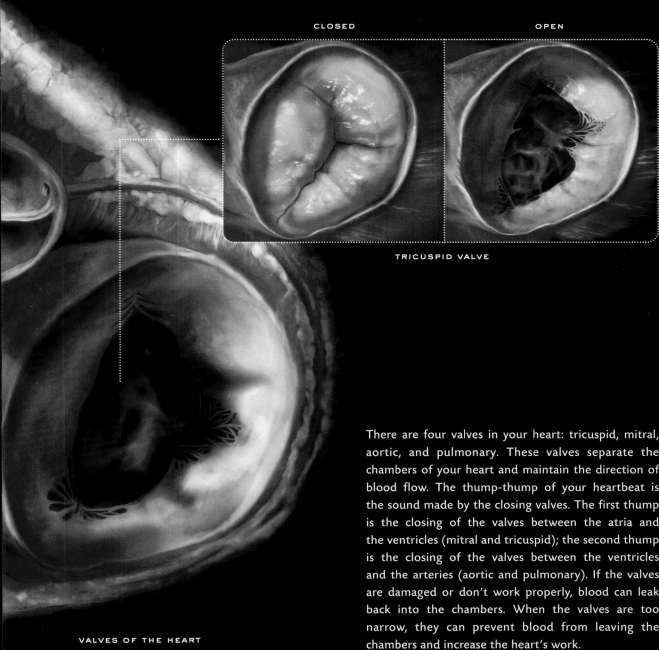

CLOSED

OPEN

TRICUSPID VALVE

VALVES OF THE HEART

There are four valves in your heart: tricuspid, mitral, aortic, and pulmonary. These valves separate the chambers of your heart and maintain the direction of blood flow. The thump-thump of your heartbeat is the sound made by the closing valves. The first thump is the closing of the valves between the atria and the ventricles (mitral and tricuspid); the second thump is the closing of the valves between the ventricles and the arteries (aortic and pulmonary). If the valves are damaged or don't work properly, blood can leak back into the chambers. When the valves are too narrow, they can prevent blood from leaving the chambers and increase the heart's work.

AN ELECTROCARDIOGRAM
(ECG) IS A MEASUREMENT
OF THE ELECTRICAL
SIGNALS OF THE HEART

CONDUCTION
SYSTEM OF
THE HEART

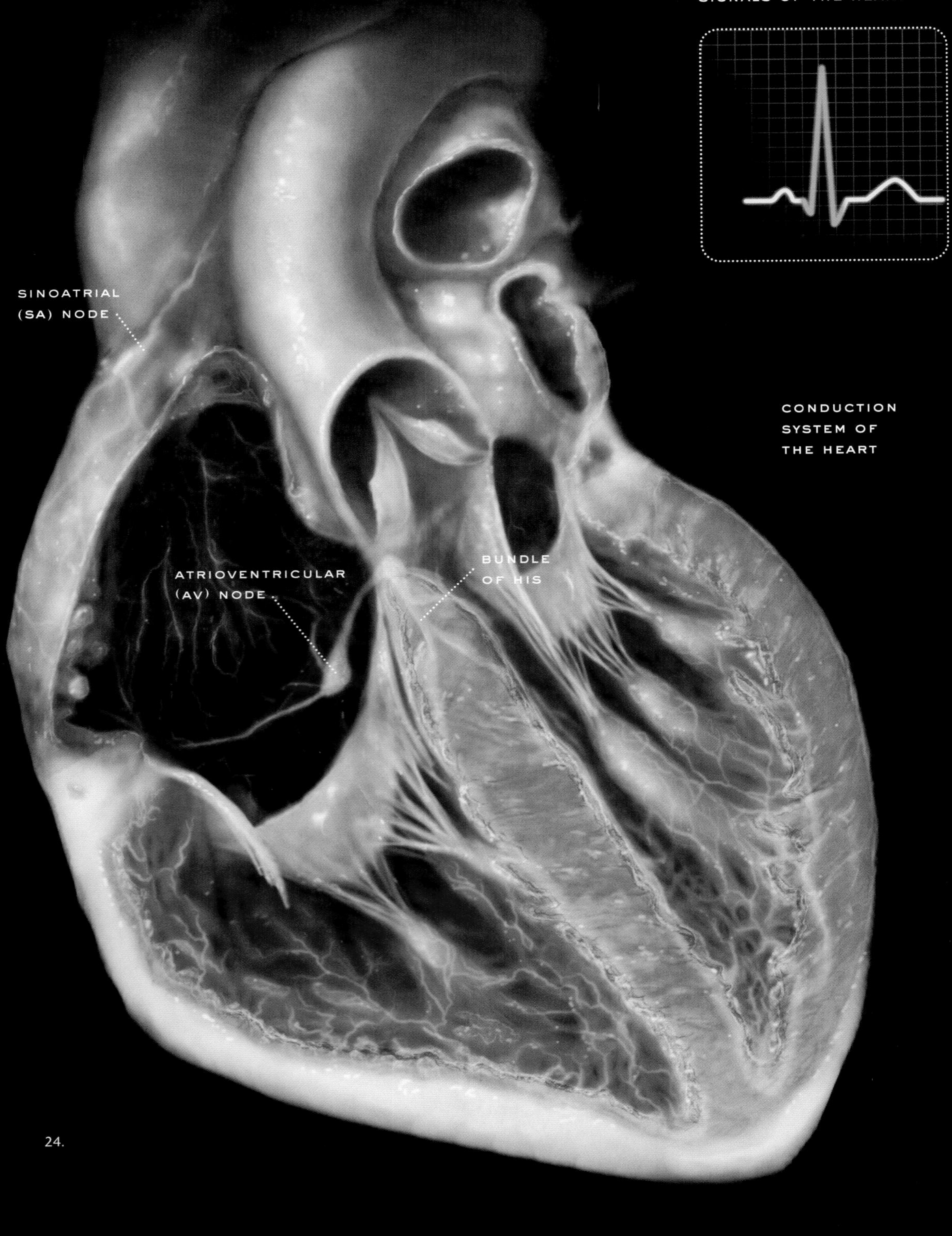

SINOATRIAL
(SA) NODE

ATRIOVENTRICULAR
(AV) NODE

BUNDLE
OF HIS

Dr. Oz has been practicing for over ten years, yet he still remembers the wonder he felt when he first began to do his job. "It's a very intimidating thing for a young surgeon to face the heart. It looks like a boa constrictor that was wrestled into this small chest cavity and it wants to get out. One of the spookiest things about heart cells is that they are powered by a mind of their own, the pacemaker cells. And so even when we do heart transplants and literally cut the heart out of the body, it keeps beating. It's an amazing thing to see."

MITOCHONDRIA (AQUA) ARE CELLULAR ORGANELLES THAT PROVIDE ENERGY TO THE MUSCLE FIBERS (PINK), WHICH ARE MADE UP OF FILAMENTS. THESE FILAMENTS SLIDE OVER ONE ANOTHER TO CONTRACT CARDIAC MUSCLE DURING A HEARTBEAT.

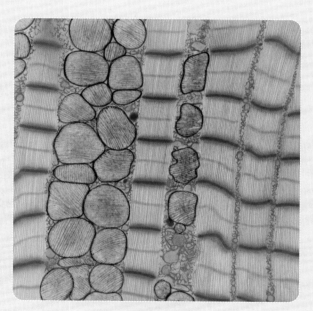

HEALTHY HEART CELLS

Your heart beats faster or slower depending on information from your brain, which monitors your body's need for blood. However, the basic rhythm of your heart is automatic; it does not depend on signals from your brain.

Your heart cells can generate their own electrical signals, which trigger the contractions and cause the entire heart to pump in synchrony. A specialized bundle of muscle and nerve cells called the sinoatrial node (SA node) sits at the top of the right atrium and is the pacemaker of the heart. It generates the signal for the atria to contract and send blood to the ventricles. A similar node—the atrioventricular or AV node—sits at the atrioventricular septum near the bottom of the right atrium and relays the signal from the SA node to the ventricles to contract and pump blood out of the heart. An electrocardiogram (ECG) measures the electrical signals given off by these two nodes and their conduction through the heart. By looking at the frequency and the height of the peaks and valleys of these signals on an ECG, healthcare professionals get a very good idea of how well the electrical system of your heart is working.

Your blood vessels also respond to the needs of your body. In addition to being the blood supply lines, blood vessels can contract or dilate to divert blood flow to different parts of the body. There are three main types of blood vessels: arteries, veins, and capillaries. At any one time, a healthy adult has about five quarts of blood moving through these vessels.

Arteries are blood vessels that carry blood away from your heart to the rest of the body and to the lungs. All arteries carry oxygenated blood except the pulmonary artery. The pulmonary artery carries deoxygenated blood from your heart to the lungs.

Veins carry blood to the heart. In general, your veins carry deoxygenated blood, but as in the arteries, the pulmonary vein is an exception. It carries oxygenated blood from the lungs back to the heart.

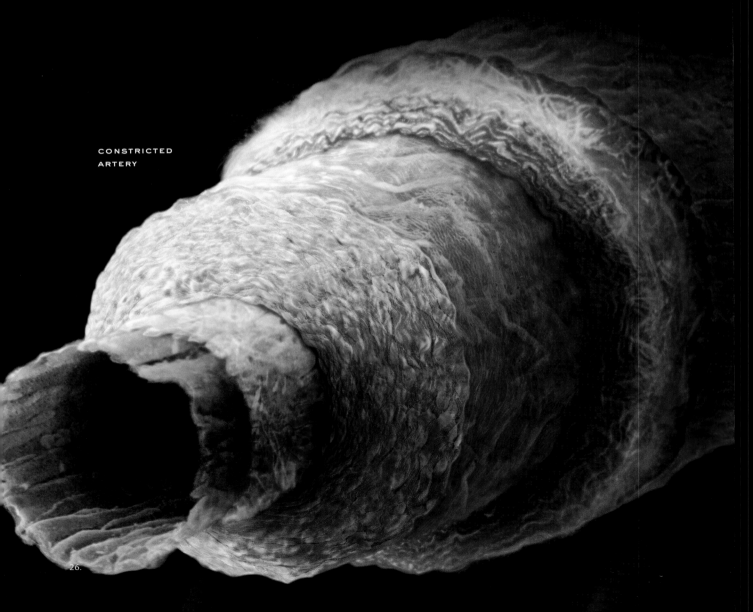

CONSTRICTED
ARTERY

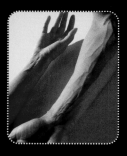

It's not just the heart Dr. Oz works on: "One of the first things I noticed as a heart surgeon was how different the arteries of women and men were. We lump men and women together in thinking of heart disease as the same ailment in both genders, but it's not; it's very different. Only 30% of women with heart problems have hardening of the arteries compared to 90% of men. The arteries of men are like linguini: they're big structures; they're easier to work with, which is why we are so much more successful when we do bypass grafts or stents on men. Women have arteries like capellini; they are really thin, small vessels."

DILATED ARTERY

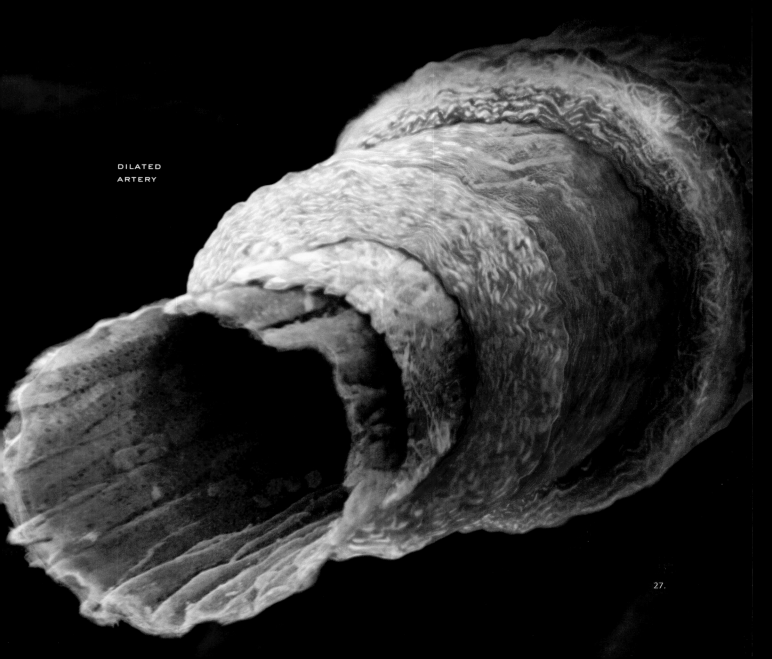

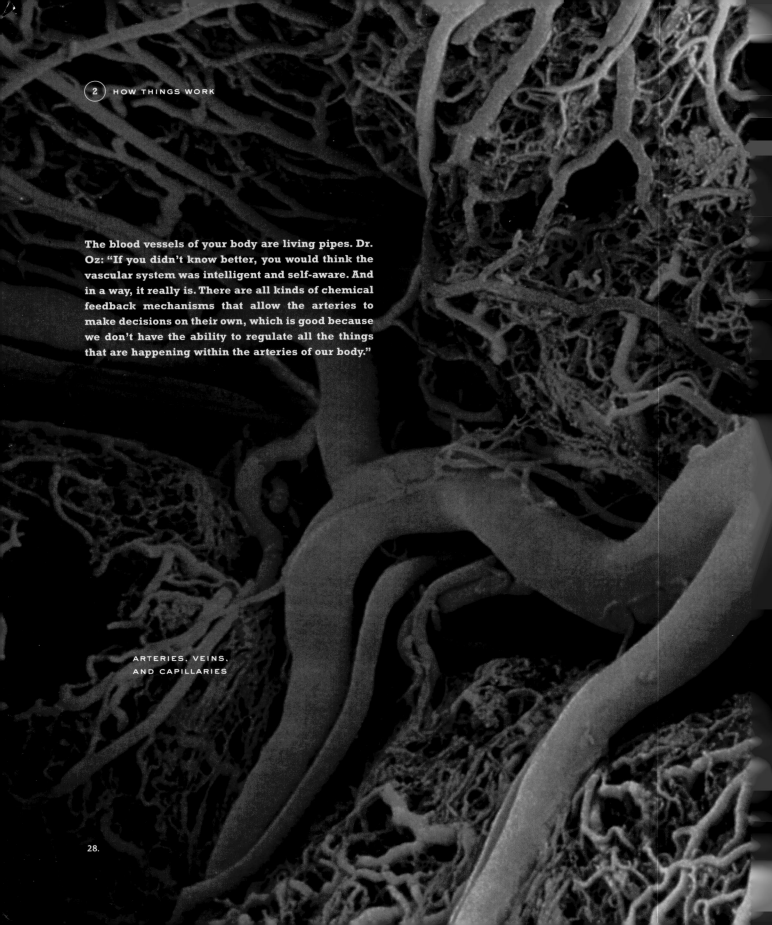

The blood vessels of your body are living pipes. Dr. Oz: "If you didn't know better, you would think the vascular system was intelligent and self-aware. And in a way, it really is. There are all kinds of chemical feedback mechanisms that allow the arteries to make decisions on their own, which is good because we don't have the ability to regulate all the things that are happening within the arteries of our body."

ARTERIES, VEINS, AND CAPILLARIES

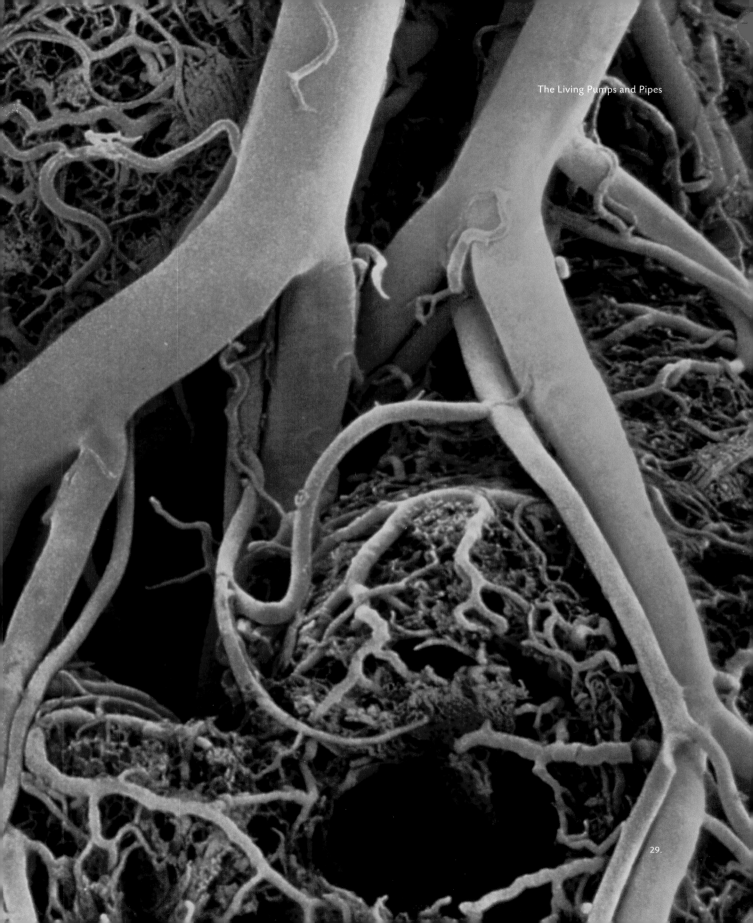

29.

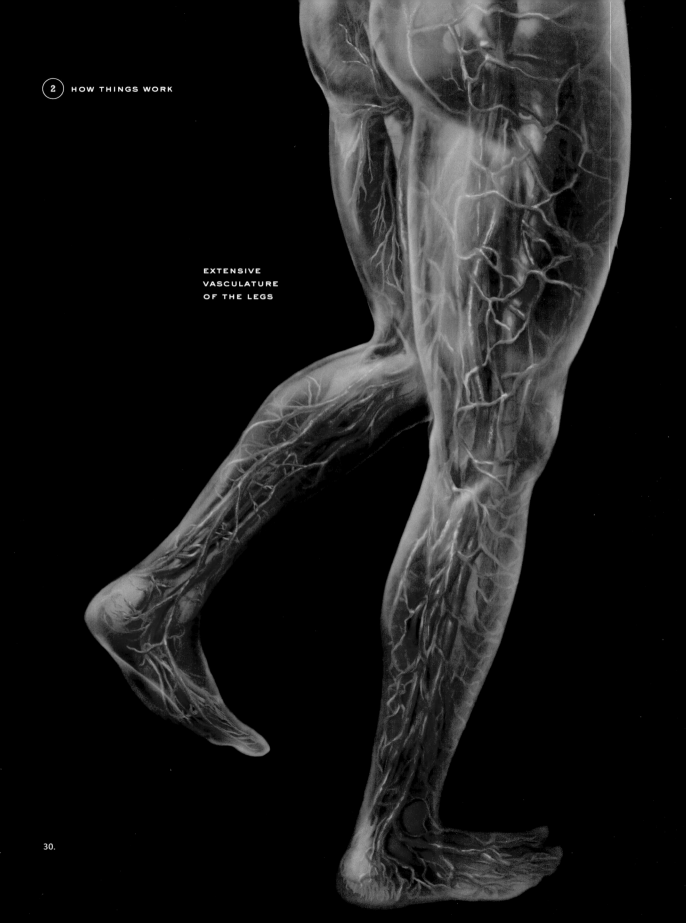

EXTENSIVE
VASCULATURE
OF THE LEGS

Your arteries are made up of three layers of cells: the *tunica intima*, the *tunica media*, and the *tunica adventitia*. The *tunica intima* is actually a single layer of endothelial cells. These cells are used as lining in many parts of your body. They provide a smooth surface for the blood to flow on. In addition, the endothelial layer is a functioning system that secretes different products and responds to different stimuli from the blood vessels and tissues.

The *tunica media* or middle layer of the artery contains the muscle cells and other structural and elastic fibers that contract and dilate the artery. One of the signs of arterial aging is a loss of the pliability of the muscle cells in the *tunica media* and a loss of ability to distend. The *tunica adventitia*, the outer layer, contains the artery's support system—tiny blood vessels that feed the artery, and nerves that respond to signals and control the artery's contraction and dilation.

Like arteries, veins are also made of three layers. However, veins do not contract like arteries. Veins in the lower part of your body have one-way valves to counteract the effects of gravity and prevent blood from flowing back into the feet. Veins in the upper part of the body have no valves because gravity itself brings the blood back down to the heart. Unfortunately, valves can be damaged and weakened over time. Varicose veins are caused by leaky valves that allow blood to pool and bulge in the veins of the legs.

Unlike arteries and veins, capillaries are made of a single layer of endothelial cells. Scattered throughout the capillary is a second type of cell called pericytes. These are smooth muscle-like cells that provide the capillary with the ability to contract. They also help feed the capillaries and control the exchange of nutrients and wastes.

ARTERY

VEIN

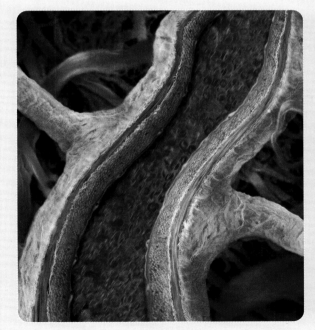
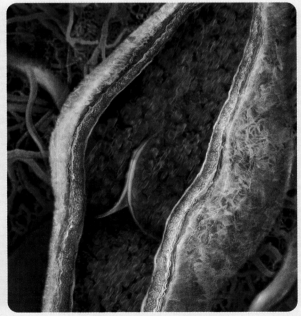

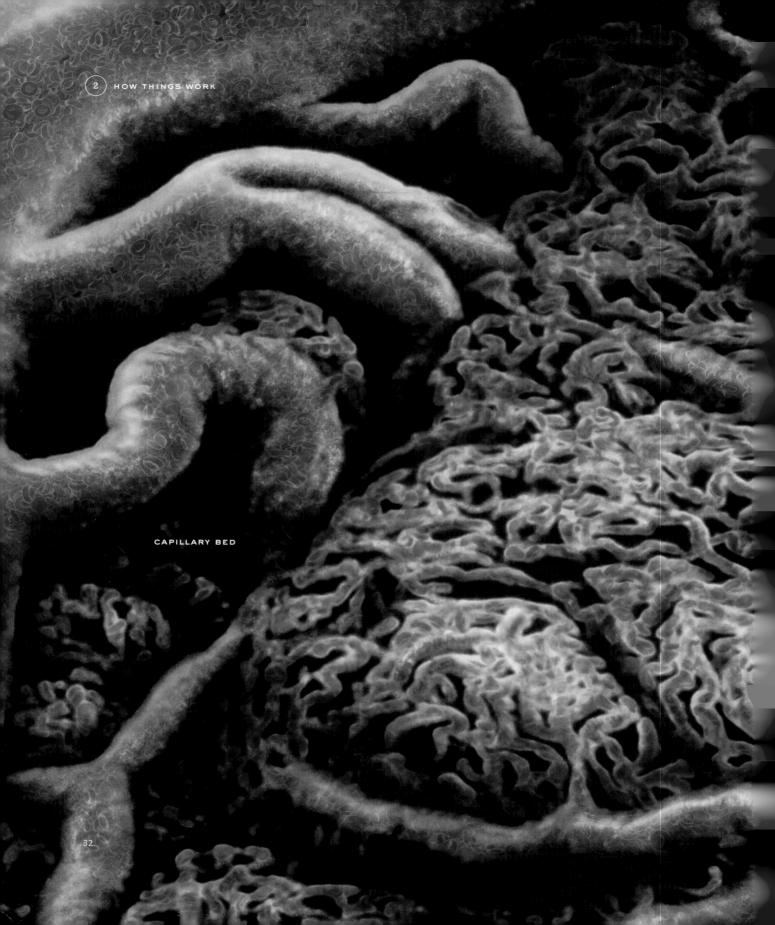

CAPILLARY BED

Over 99% of the blood vessels in your body are capillaries, even though they hold less than 5% of your blood. The capillaries are so extensive that each cell of your body is within reach of one. Proximity to cells is important. These tiny blood vessels are the key sites for exchanges of nutrients and wastes. In general, nutrients flow out of the capillary to the cells, and waste products flow from the cells into the capillaries.

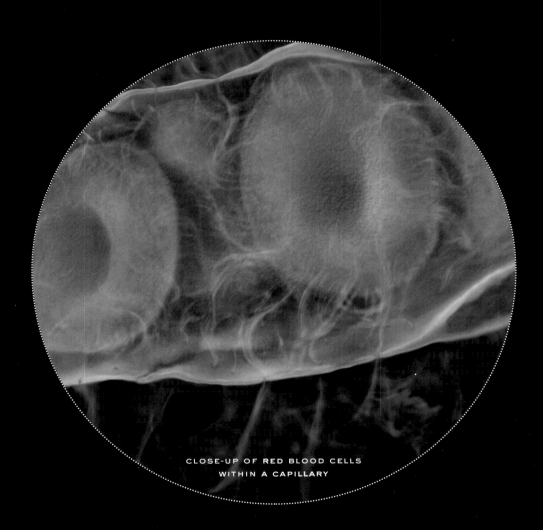

CLOSE-UP OF RED BLOOD CELLS
WITHIN A CAPILLARY

The cardiovascular system is an integrated network from the largest vessels to the smallest. Dr. Oz: "There are dozens of major arteries and millions of smaller ones that carry the blood supply to the tissues where the energy is needed. And it's on the subtlety of the function of those small vessels where most disease focuses."

However, the capillaries that carry the blood supply to the kidneys and intestines act differently. The role of the kidneys is to filter wastes out of the blood for disposal. Filtration is a multistep process. Glomeruli—ball-shaped bundles of capillaries—are the filtering units of the kidney. High pressure forces out fluid and small waste products through slits in the capillaries within the glomeruli. The slits are too small to let blood cells and large molecules pass through; these are kept for later recycling. Thus, the pressure in the glomeruli remains high, as there is little to no resorption from the surrounding cells. In contrast, the main role of the intestines is to provide nutrients to the body. The surrounding capillaries are at relatively low pressure, which allows nutrients to flow into the circulatory system with little filtration back into the intestines.

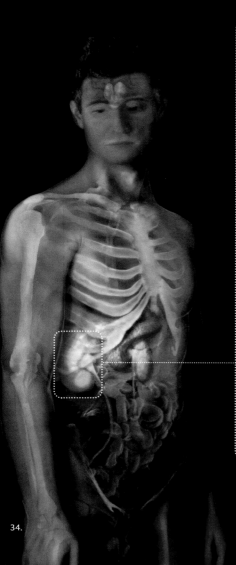

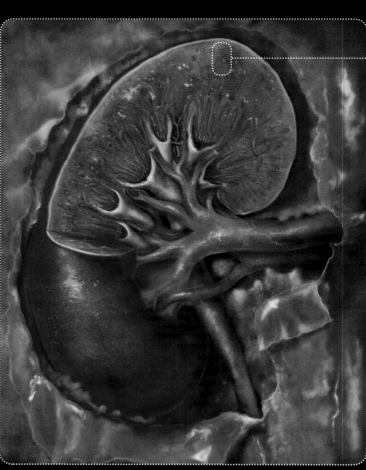

KIDNEY

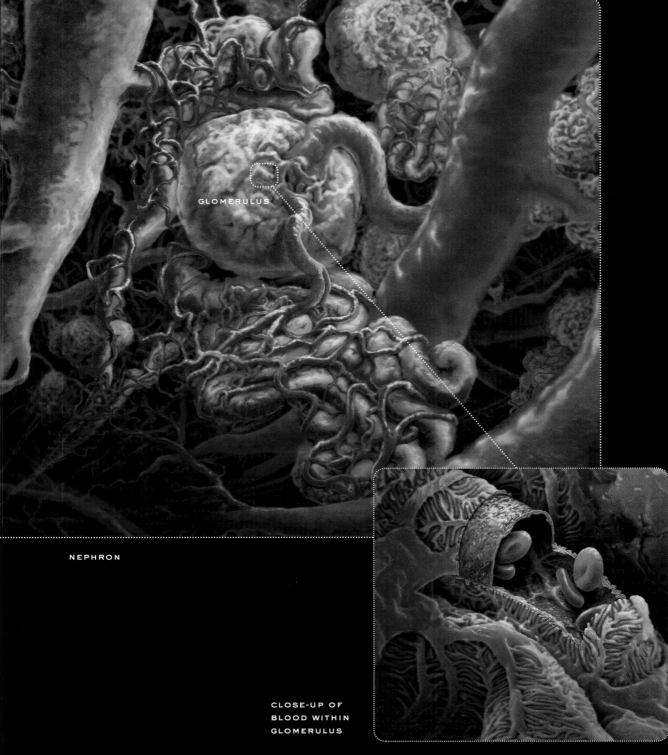

GLOMERULUS

NEPHRON

CLOSE-UP OF
BLOOD WITHIN
GLOMERULUS

35.

The pulmonary circulation and systemic circulation are tied together in that they work in synchrony to provide the body with oxygen and to get rid of the body's carbon dioxide. Enzymes digest, or break down, the carbohydrates from the foods you eat into sugars, which the cells of your body use to produce energy. Oxygen is needed for energy production, and carbon dioxide is one of the waste products. These gases are transported by your cardiovascular system through the blood.

Your blood has cells called red blood cells, or erythrocytes. These cells have molecules (hemoglobin), which can bind to or release oxygen as needed. When you breathe, oxygenated air flows through your lungs and ends up in thousands of small air sacs in the lungs called alveoli. The right side of your heart sends deoxygenated blood to the capillaries surrounding these alveoli. The walls between the alveoli and the capillaries are extremely thin, so that the inhaled oxygen can seep from the air sacs to bind to the hemoglobin molecules in the erythrocytes. Carbon dioxide and other waste gases leave the blood and diffuse into the air sacs, where they are exhaled through the lungs. This gas exchange is passive: oxygen goes from the higher concentration in the lungs to the lower concentration in the blood. Similarly, carbon dioxide goes from the blood to the lungs.

TRANSPARENT LUNGS
REVEALING AIRWAYS
AND BLOOD VESSELS

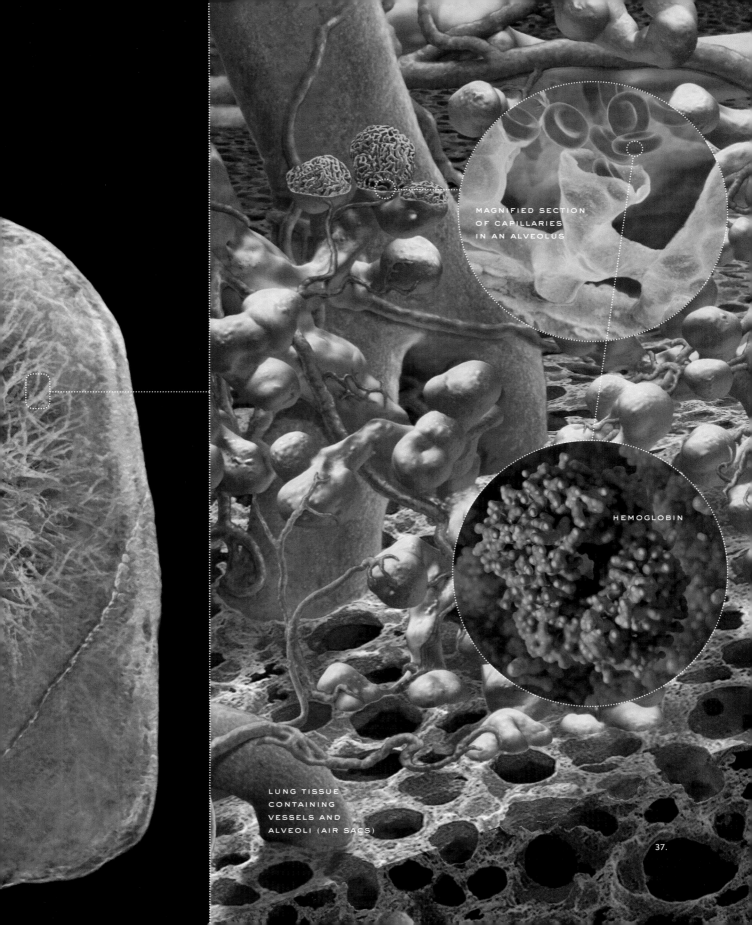

MAGNIFIED SECTION
OF CAPILLARIES
IN AN ALVEOLUS

HEMOGLOBIN

LUNG TISSUE
CONTAINING
VESSELS AND
ALVEOLI (AIR SACS)

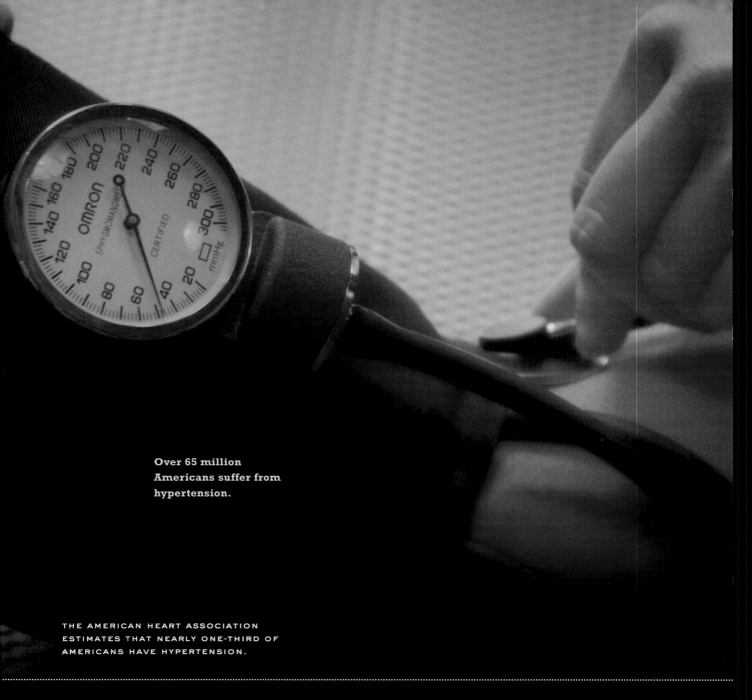

Over 65 million
Americans suffer from
hypertension.

THE AMERICAN HEART ASSOCIATION
ESTIMATES THAT NEARLY ONE-THIRD OF
AMERICANS HAVE HYPERTENSION.

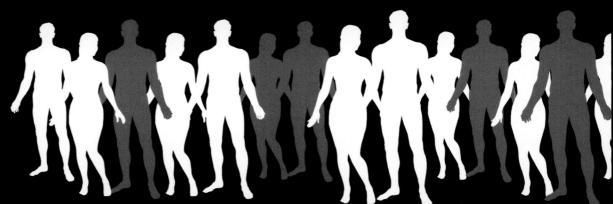

WHEN YOUR HEART BEATS, IT IS LITERALLY FORCING BLOOD THROUGH THE VESSELS TO REACH ALL PARTS OF THE BODY. BLOOD PRESSURE—THE AMOUNT OF FORCE THE BLOOD EXERTS ON THE VESSEL WALLS—IS THUS A MEASURE OF THE HEALTH OF THE CARDIOVASCULAR SYSTEM. A SIMPLE, QUICK, PAINLESS PROCEDURE INVOLVING A PRESSURE CUFF AND GAUGE GIVES THE TWO NUMBERS IN A BLOOD PRESSURE READING.

CHAPTER

3

when things go wrong:
grace under pressure

One of the main indicators (and causes) of cardiovascular disease is high blood pressure (hypertension). Hypertension is caused by many factors: Genetic disposition, age, gender, the history of other diseases, lifestyle choices, all play a part in a person's risk and the severity of the disease. Hypertension may have no initial symptoms, but over 65 million Americans suffer its damaging effects. Some 15 million people don't even know they have high blood pressure. They don't know that with every beat of their heart, they're risking heart failure, strokes, and other types of cardiovascular damage.

GRACE IS A COMPOSITE CHARACTER WHO HAS THE TYPICAL CHARACTERISTICS OF A PATIENT WITH HIGH BLOOD PRESSURE.

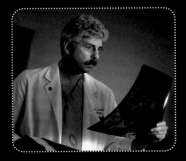

Cardiologists like Peter Fail, M.D., are on the front lines of a growing crisis in America. At the Cardiovascular Institute of the South in Houma, Louisiana, many of Dr. Fail's patients have sky-high blood pressure readings. Grace, a 45-year-old mother of two, is one such patient. Her blood pressure is 150/100. Dr. Fail says: "People think that it's okay to have high blood pressure if they have a reason for it. I had a fight with my husband this morning, so it's okay for me to have high blood pressure. I have a high-stress job and therefore it's okay for me to have high blood pressure. But it's not okay; the stroke that's going to be caused by the high blood pressure doesn't care."

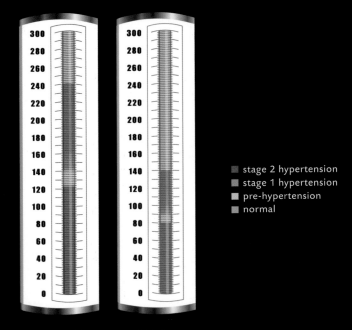

■ stage 2 hypertension
■ stage 1 hypertension
■ pre-hypertension
■ normal

SYSTOLIC   DIASTOLIC

The first of the two numbers in a blood pressure reading (systolic) is the force on the arterial wall generated by the heart pumping out blood. The second number (diastolic) is the force when the heart is filling with blood. A healthy adult blood pressure reading is 120/80 or below. For every increase of 20 in the systolic number or 10 in the diastolic, the cardiovascular risk doubles. Even people with a blood pressure reading only slightly above normal— prehypertensives—may be on the road to poor cardiovascular health.

Many factors influence the pressure in the cardiovascular system. Water, salt, food intake, outside temperature, and level of activity all have a huge impact on the volume of blood, its thickness, and the speed of flow. Yet a healthy cardiovascular system adapts within seconds to different stimuli to adjust the pressure.

40.

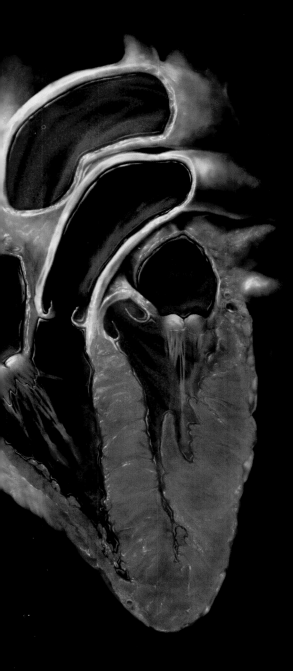

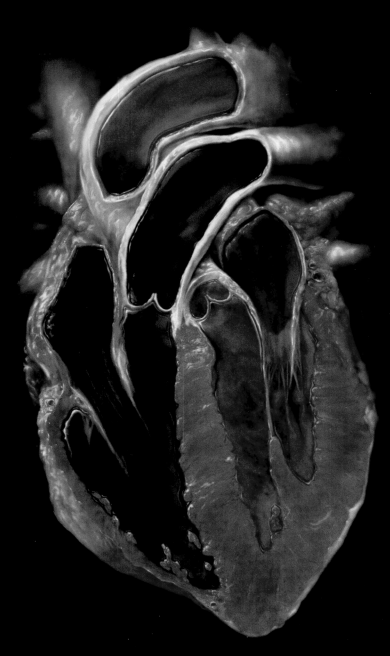

DURING SYSTOLE, THE VENTRICLES CONTRACT TO SQUEEZE BLOOD OUT TO THE REST OF THE BODY.

DURING DIASTOLE, THE VENTRICLES DILATE TO ALLOW THE BLOOD TO FILL THE HEART.

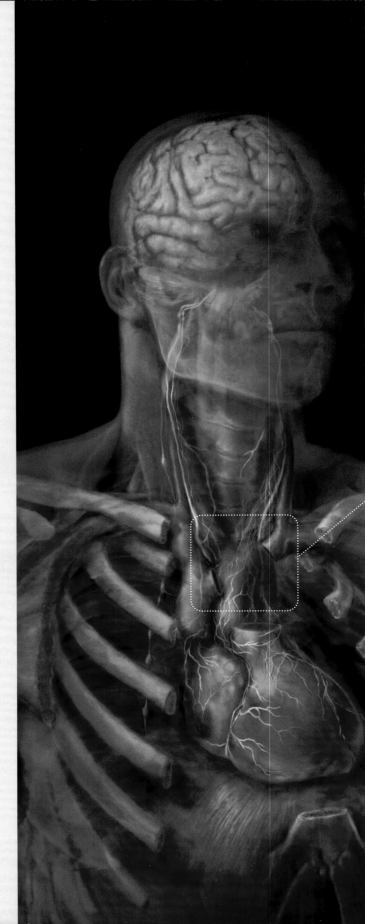

The most obvious way in which your body manages blood flow and pressure is to change the heart rate. In general, when the pulse rate goes up, the pressure in the system goes up, which in turn drives the blood around the body more quickly. The blood vessels themselves also play an important role in pressure management. Blood vessels are living pipes. They're elastic and flexible and have special sensors called baroreceptors that monitor the ebb and flow of blood. Baroreceptors are actually nerve bundles that provide immediate feedback to the brain. With this information and depending on the needs of the moment, the arteries dilate and contract to help propel blood through the system. Blood can be diverted to muscles during exercise, for example, or away from the skin during cold weather to avoid heat loss. The arteries can contract to prevent blood loss due to injury or dilate to flood the face for that telling blush.

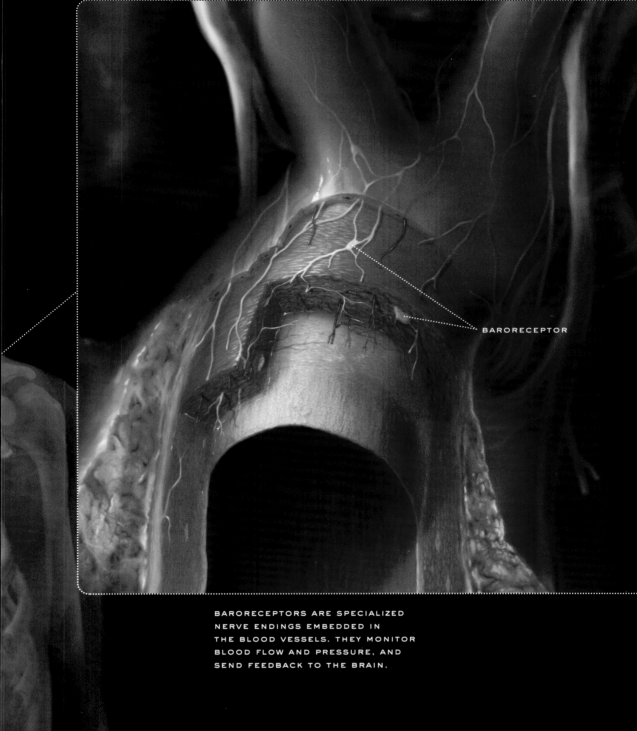

BARORECEPTOR

BARORECEPTORS ARE SPECIALIZED
NERVE ENDINGS EMBEDDED IN
THE BLOOD VESSELS. THEY MONITOR
BLOOD FLOW AND PRESSURE, AND
SEND FEEDBACK TO THE BRAIN.

Grace is overweight. The typical Cajun diet has had a detrimental effect on her blood pressure and the condition of her blood vessels. "South Louisiana is known for its food," says Dr. Fail. "It's absolutely some of the best food in the world. Unfortunately, it's also probably the least heart-healthy food in the world. They will fry absolutely everything down here. And that's a problem. It becomes a little bit more difficult to try and convince the Cajun population here to eat healthier, to get away from a high-fat diet and try to incorporate more of the low-fat options—the vegetables and the fruits. Our food is one of the things that's killing us slowly but surely."

HEALTHY BLOOD VESSELS
ARE SMOOTH AND FLEXIBLE.

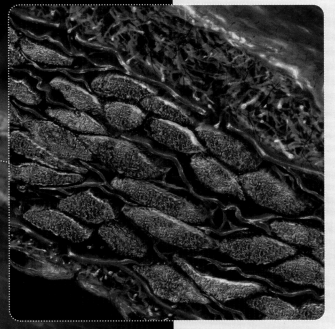

In a healthy body, the blood vessels are smooth and elastic. As we age, the stretchy elastic fibers in the vessel walls are replaced with less flexible material. This stiffer material—collagen—makes the blood vessels less able to expand. High blood pressure puts additional stress on the vessel walls and accelerates this hardening process.

As blood rushes through these stiffer vessels, the pressure rises. The heart has to work harder to pump blood through the unyielding stiff vessels, and in doing so the pressure rises. In general, the lower the pressure the better: even pressure readings of 130/80 can lead to heart attacks. The American Society of Hypertension, Inc. classifies any reading of 140/90 and above as hypertension and a condition that must be treated.

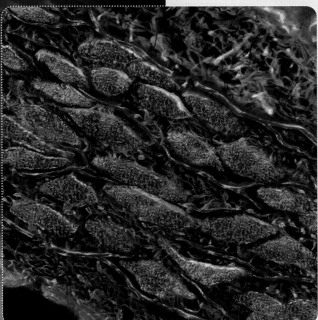

UNHEALTHY BLOOD VESSELS
ARE STIFF AND RIGID.

Grace came to see her doctor because she has been feeling tired and finds it harder to catch her breath. Not all patients with hypertension have symptoms. Many have no idea of the danger they're in. Dr. Fail observes: "High pressure hurts organs; like a blast from a fire hose."

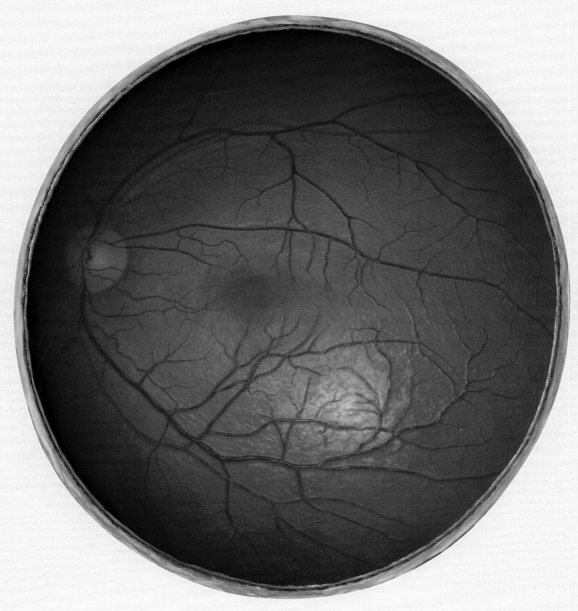

HEALTHY RETINA

Your body works best under a defined set of parameters. High blood pressure exceeds these parameters and thus damages other parts of the body.

Your eyes are particularly susceptible. Capillaries—the smallest type of blood vessels—supply blood to the retina, the part of the eye that receives visual images. In patients with hypertension, the pressure can burst these fragile capillaries and blood can leak into the retina. In extremely advanced cases of hypertension, this can cause problems with vision and blindness.

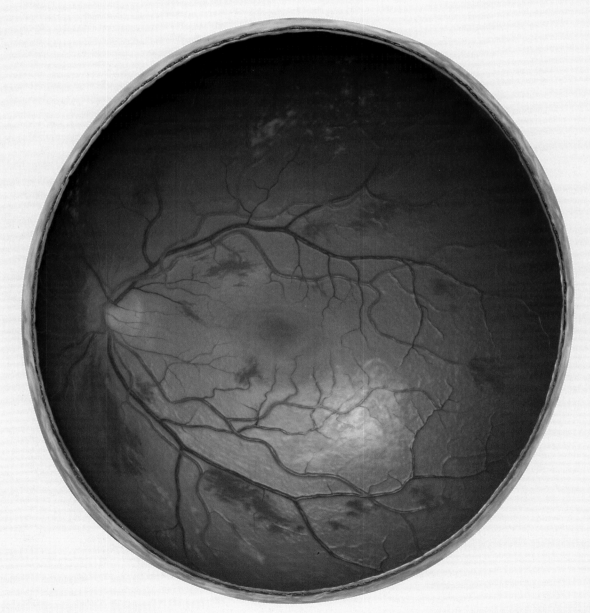

UNHEALTHY RETINA REVEALING CAPILLARY
DAMAGE CAUSED BY HYPERTENSION

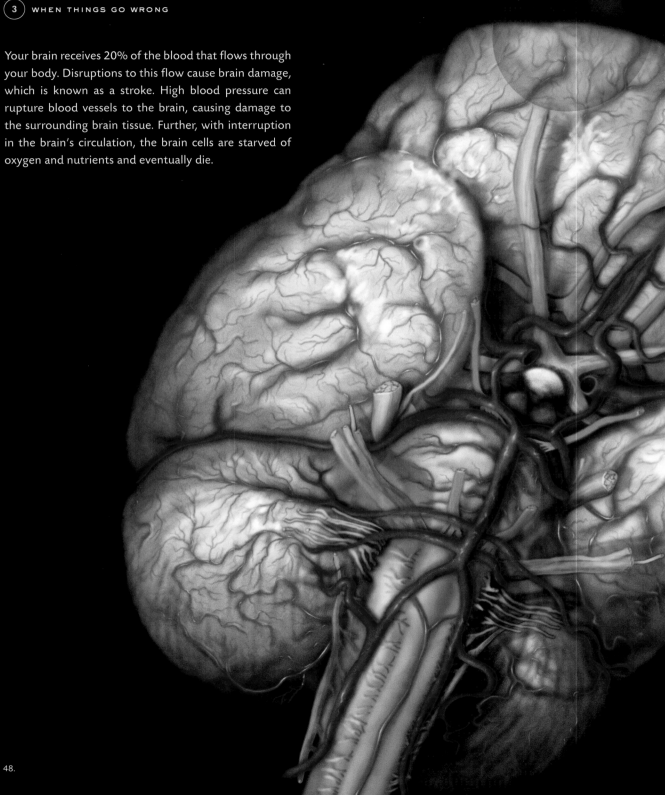

Your brain receives 20% of the blood that flows through your body. Disruptions to this flow cause brain damage, which is known as a stroke. High blood pressure can rupture blood vessels to the brain, causing damage to the surrounding brain tissue. Further, with interruption in the brain's circulation, the brain cells are starved of oxygen and nutrients and eventually die.

VIEW OF THE BASE OF
A HYPERTENSIVE BRAIN

HIGH BLOOD PRESSURE CAN
RUPTURE BLOOD VESSELS IN
THE BRAIN, CAUSING DAMAGE
TO SURROUNDING TISSUE.

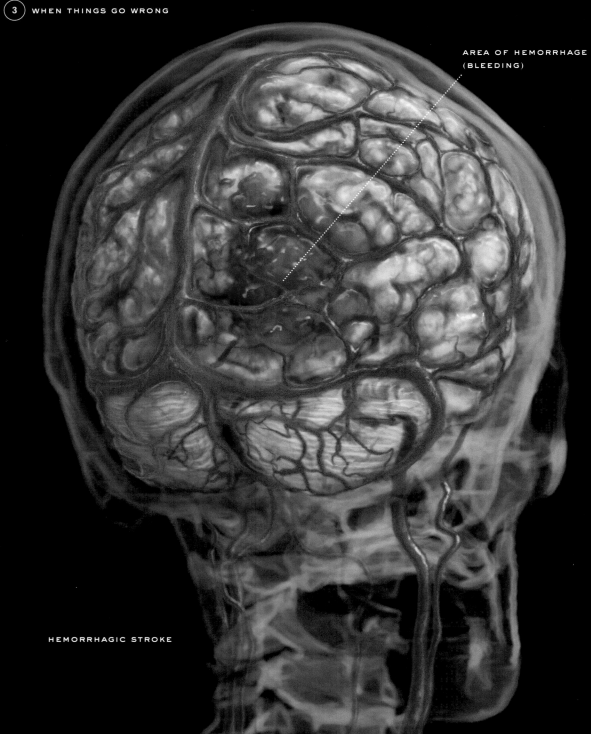

AREA OF HEMORRHAGE
(BLEEDING)

HEMORRHAGIC STROKE

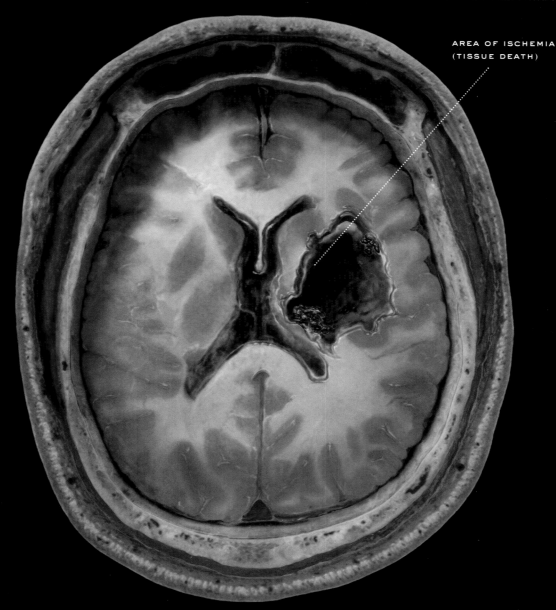

AREA OF ISCHEMIA
(TISSUE DEATH)

ISCHEMIC STROKE

Bleeding, or hemorrhagic strokes are relatively uncommon but deadly: half the people who have a hemorrhagic stroke die. The other type of stroke—ischemic—is caused by a blood clot or a narrowing of the arteries. A cholesterol-containing fatty substance called plaque can build up and coat the inside of vessels, decreasing their diameter and thus blood flow. Blood clots that build on top of plaque deposits can loosen and break off and then clog smaller blood vessels, disrupting blood flow.

PLAQUE STARTS TO COAT THE INSIDE OF A VESSEL.

PLAQUE BUILDUP ACCELERATES.

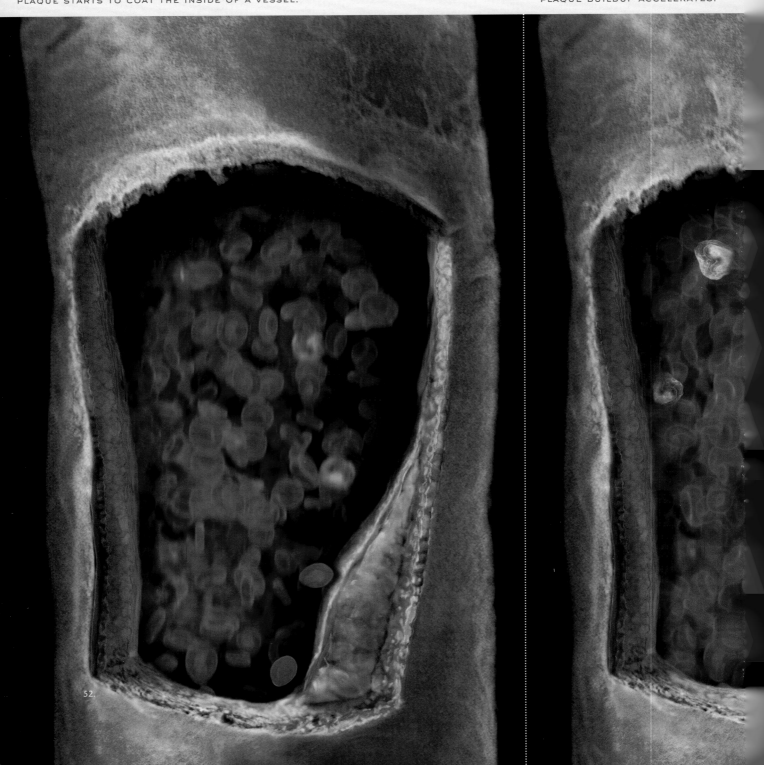

52.

PLAQUE RUPTURE CAN CAUSE CLOTS THAT CAN BREAK OFF
AND BLOCK BLOOD FLOW IN A SMALLER VESSEL.

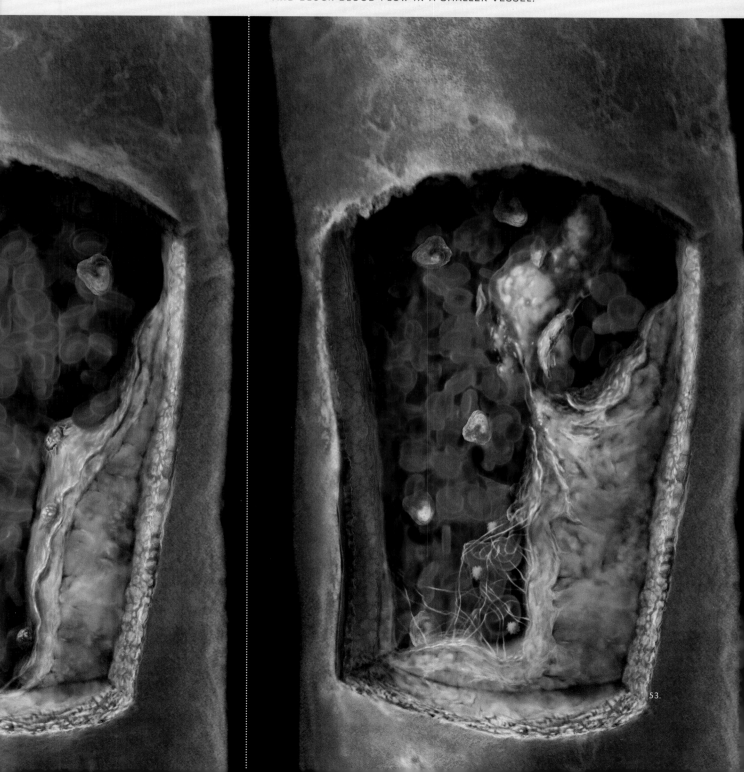

53.

Grace's kidneys are still working well; however, others with hypertension are not so lucky. People with chronic kidney disease often suffer from hypertension and vice versa. Kidney failure means dialysis—three times a week, for four hours at a time. Karol Watson, M.D., is the co-director of the UCLA Program in Preventative Cardiology in Los Angeles. Many of her patients have kidney problems. Dr. Watson notes, "What your kidneys were able to do is now being done by a machine. All the blood in your body is passed through a machine, cleaned, and then passed back into the body. Dialysis is lifesaving, but it is also life-altering."

Your kidneys are responsible for the level of dissolved salt in the blood, which affects the thickness or viscosity of the blood. Even more importantly, your kidneys remove excess salt and water from your system, which in turn determines the volume of blood in the body and hence its pressure. In fact, when receptors in the heart detect an excess of blood pressure, they immediately send chemical messengers to the kidneys with instructions to remove more water and salt from the blood.

High blood pressure damages the arteries and the tiny blood vessels in the kidneys where filtration occurs. This sets up a vicious cycle where the weakened kidneys are less able to filter blood, which means blood volume and viscosity are harder to control, thus escalating the damage to the cardiovascular system. Indeed, the link between high blood pressure and impaired kidney function is so close that patients who receive kidney transplants often see their high blood pressure improve.

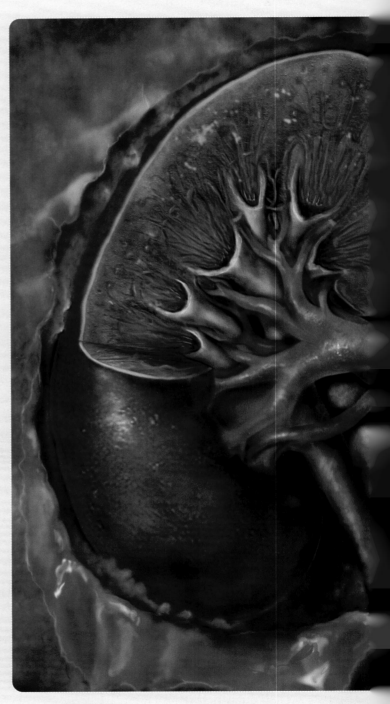

NORMAL KIDNEY

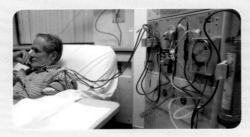

PATIENT ON DIALYSIS

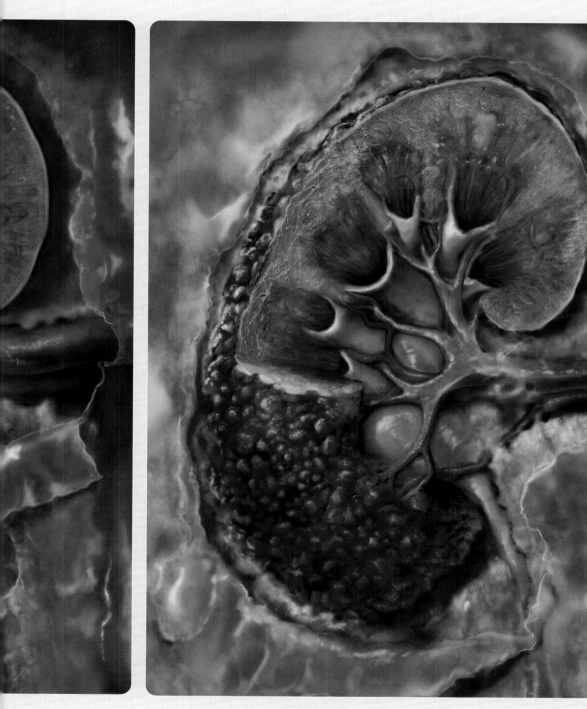

UNHEALTHY KIDNEY REVEALING VESSEL AND TISSUE
DAMAGE CAUSED BY HIGH BLOOD PRESSURE

For some people with hypertension, telling them that they're big-hearted is not good news. Dr. Fail: "I tell my patients to think of it as a rubber band. You put one rubber band on and you can work that rubber band very nicely and that would be a normal heart. And if you put two or three or four rubber bands on, you can't relax, the heart won't relax. Well, that's what happens when the heart muscle gets thick: it doesn't relax. And it's just as bad as if that rubber band didn't come together, if it's lost its elasticity; that also becomes a problem. High blood pressure can harm many organs in the body; but some of the worst damage happens right at the center of the cardiovascular system, in the heart itself. Overgrowth of the left ventricle, or left ventricular hypertrophy (LVH), is a significant effect of high blood pressure."

Your heart is the strongest muscle in the body; however, like any other muscle, the harder it works, the bigger it gets. In individuals with high blood pressure, where vessels are damaged and stiff, the heart is forced to pump harder with each beat to push blood out into the system. At first, the increase in size allows the heart to pump harder, but over time, the ventricle walls stretch, then thicken and grow stiff. The result is a heart that is both bigger and weaker.

NORMAL HEART

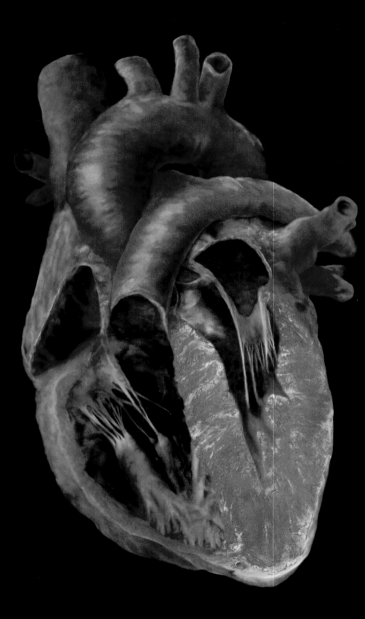

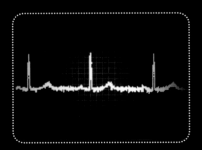

ECG: NORMAL HEARTBEAT

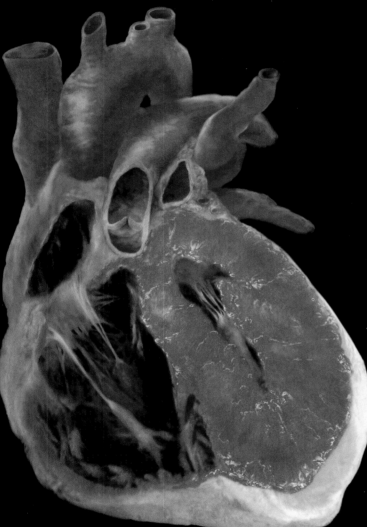

ENLARGED HEART

As Dr. Fail suspected, high blood pressure has taken its toll. Grace's heart is enlarged. Without treatment, Grace is in danger of heart failure.

As the muscle tissue in an overstressed heart expands, blood supply to the heart muscle is lost, resulting in damage to the heart. To maintain blood supply to the body, the heart remodels—fibrous tissues or scars are formed. The scar tissue is hard and cannot conduct electricity well from cell to cell. The result is that the system can no longer be relied on to deliver the carefully synchronized pattern of jolts needed to keep the heart pumping smoothly. This condition is called arrhythmia.

In some cases, arrhythmia can mean simply that the heartbeat is too fast or too slow—a bothersome but not necessarily life-threatening condition. In the worst cases, the arrhythmia indicates a potentially lethal instability in the heart's electric system. The signals that control the heart's contractions get crossed and the heart spasms. If not corrected immediately, this fibrillation of the heart is often fatal. In the United States, more than 1,000 people die every day from sudden cardiac death, or cardiac arrest.

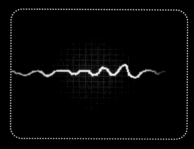

ECG: ARRHYTHMIA

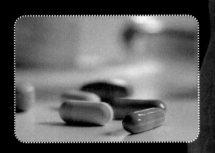

The body's blood pressure management system is extraordinarily complex. It involves several organs, billions of nerves and blood vessels, and dozens of chemical signaling systems, all working together.

Your body is a chemistry lab; it uses and produces many different molecules to carry out various functions such as blood pressure management. Angiotensin II is one molecule your body makes naturally to control salt and water balance and vessel contraction, and thus blood pressure. The cells of the brain, blood vessels, kidneys, and the heart all have receptors that respond to the levels of angiotensin II in the body. Medications that block the receptor, or prevent the action of angiotensin II, are often used to treat high blood pressure. Other types of medication affect fluid balance more directly by causing the body to excrete water and salt, thus decreasing fluid volume. These types of drugs are also used to treat people with kidney and other diseases that affect fluid balance in the body.

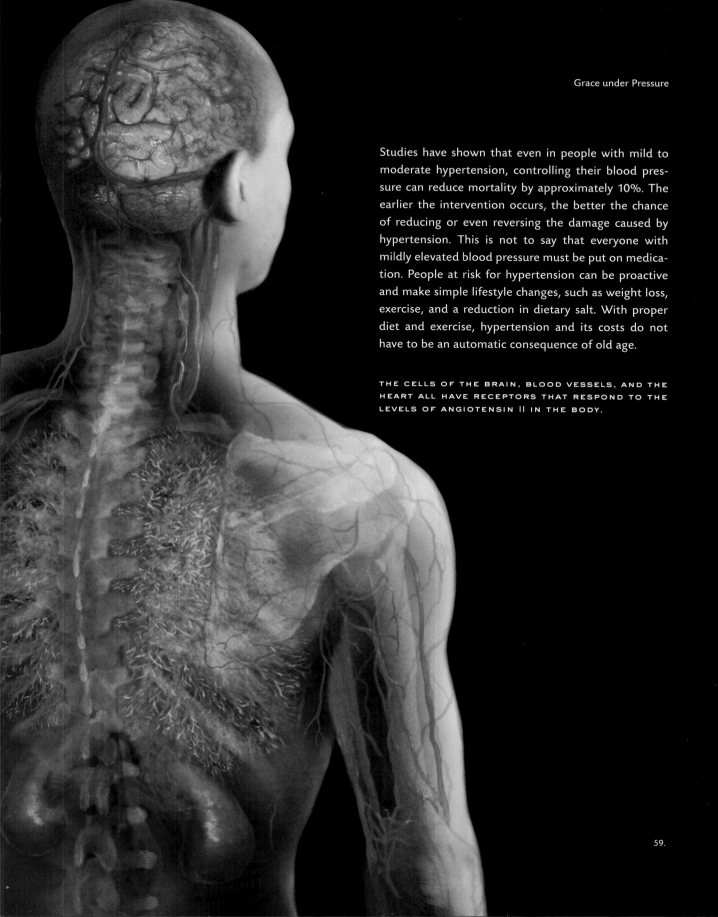

Studies have shown that even in people with mild to moderate hypertension, controlling their blood pressure can reduce mortality by approximately 10%. The earlier the intervention occurs, the better the chance of reducing or even reversing the damage caused by hypertension. This is not to say that everyone with mildly elevated blood pressure must be put on medication. People at risk for hypertension can be proactive and make simple lifestyle changes, such as weight loss, exercise, and a reduction in dietary salt. With proper diet and exercise, hypertension and its costs do not have to be an automatic consequence of old age.

THE CELLS OF THE BRAIN, BLOOD VESSELS, AND THE HEART ALL HAVE RECEPTORS THAT RESPOND TO THE LEVELS OF ANGIOTENSIN II IN THE BODY.

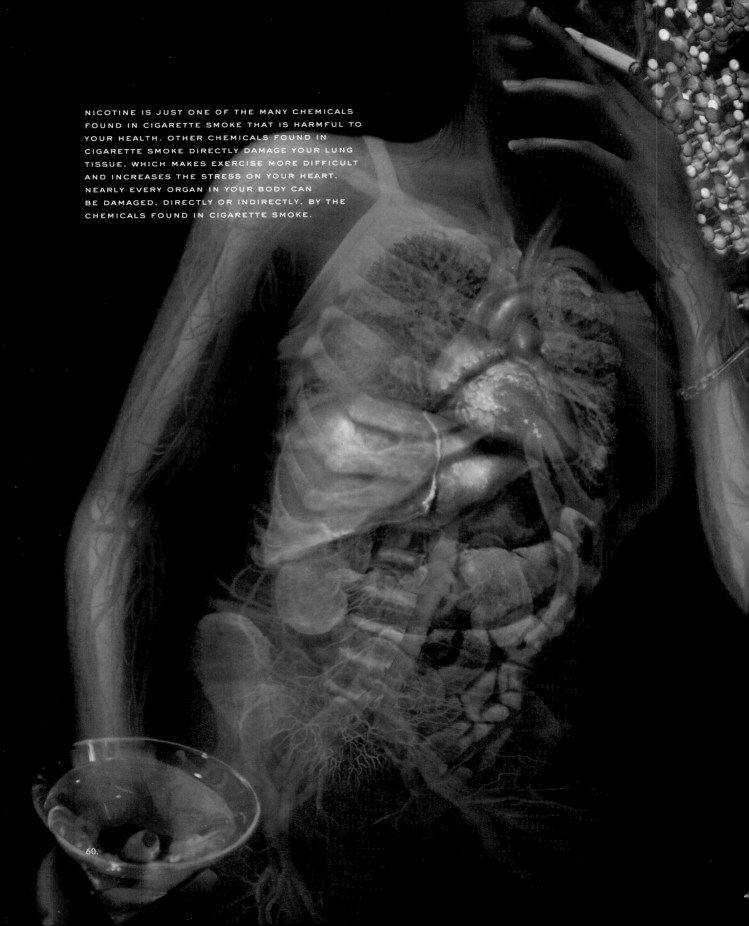

NICOTINE IS JUST ONE OF THE MANY CHEMICALS
FOUND IN CIGARETTE SMOKE THAT IS HARMFUL TO
YOUR HEALTH. OTHER CHEMICALS FOUND IN
CIGARETTE SMOKE DIRECTLY DAMAGE YOUR LUNG
TISSUE, WHICH MAKES EXERCISE MORE DIFFICULT
AND INCREASES THE STRESS ON YOUR HEART.
NEARLY EVERY ORGAN IN YOUR BODY CAN
BE DAMAGED, DIRECTLY OR INDIRECTLY, BY THE
CHEMICALS FOUND IN CIGARETTE SMOKE.

60.

DNA STRAND

CHAPTER

4

the heart of the matter: understanding the major cardiovascular risk factors

In 1948, a group of scientists began a study to see if they could discover the risk factors for heart disease. The idea was to track the health, diet, and habits of a group of people over a period of time to see what, if anything, could cause poor cardiovascular health. They recruited over 5,000 healthy people, men and women between the ages of 30 and 60 years, in the town of Framingham, Massachusetts. These people, and their children who were brought into the study 55 years later, have changed the world's understanding of cardiovascular disease.

Before the Framingham Heart Study, progressive cardiovascular disease was thought to be unavoidable. High blood pressure and arteriosclerosis (hardening of the arteries) were thought to be symptoms of an aging system. High cholesterol, a high-salt diet, and smoking were not understood as major risk factors for heart disease and other health problems. Thus, the consequences of poor cardiovascular health—heart attacks and strokes, for instance—were seen as a tragic part of the natural aging process.

Today, thanks to the results from studies like the Framingham Study, doctors can make recommendations that cut the risk of cardiovascular disease. Currently following its third generation of subjects, the Framingham Heart Study will continue to provide invaluable information on genetic, behavioral, and environmental risk factors affecting cardiovascular health.

When you look at Isobel, you see your favorite grandmother—the one who takes you on trips and goes shopping with the whole family. She's fun, happy, and independent. Recently, she had trouble keeping up with her daughters at the mall, and started to feel some pain and pressure deep in her chest. Isobel is 74, and she has been taking medication to treat her hypertension for almost ten years. Last year she was also diagnosed with low-level diabetes. She has already been warned of the complications that a condition like diabetes can add to her cardiovascular problems.

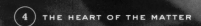

PANCREAS

KIDNEY

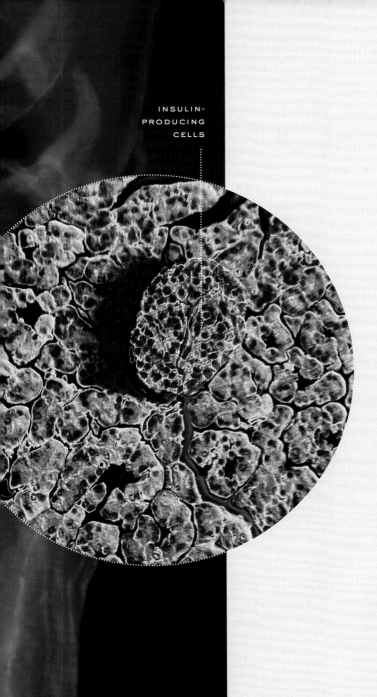

INSULIN-
PRODUCING
CELLS

Diabetes has long been linked to chronic kidney disease and other complications. The Framingham Study was able to show that diabetes also compounds cardiovascular problems. More than 20% of the population over the age of sixty-five is diabetic. Whether you have insulin dependent or non-insulin dependent diabetes, the basic problem is the same: diabetics cannot control the level of glucose (sugar) in the blood.

Sugar is one of the nutrients your body uses for energy. It is the product of the body's breakdown of complex carbohydrates and is circulated in the blood to all your cells. Although blood sugar levels change depending on whether you just ate or exercised, in general, your body keeps the sugar levels within a narrow range. Not enough sugar—hypoglycemia—and you can become hungry, shaky, sweaty, tired, and even faint. Too much sugar—hyperglycemia—is a cardiovascular risk factor leading to arteriosclerosis (hardening of the arteries). To control blood sugar levels, your body depends on a hormone called insulin.

Insulin is made by your pancreas—an organ located just behind your stomach. Insulin is a hormone that allows your cells to absorb sugar from the blood, thus lowering the sugar levels. Your cells then convert the sugars into energy or other types of molecules for storage. In diabetes, either the body produces insufficient insulin, or the cells no longer respond normally to insulin.

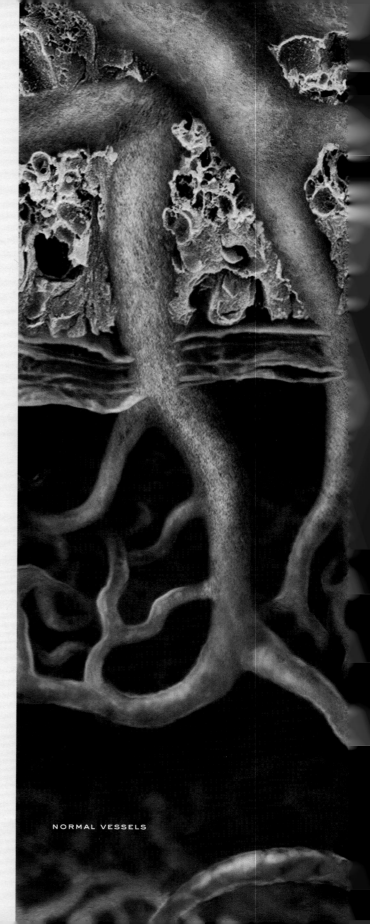

High blood sugar stresses and damages cells, especially the filtering capillaries in the kidneys and the capillaries in the back of your eyes. Thus, many diabetics suffer from chronic kidney disease, which then increases their blood pressure. Damage from the high blood sugar compounded with the increasing blood pressure can lead to vision loss. People with diabetes often also have high blood cholesterol that contributes to atherosclerosis, thereby increasing the risk of heart attacks and strokes.

NORMAL VESSELS

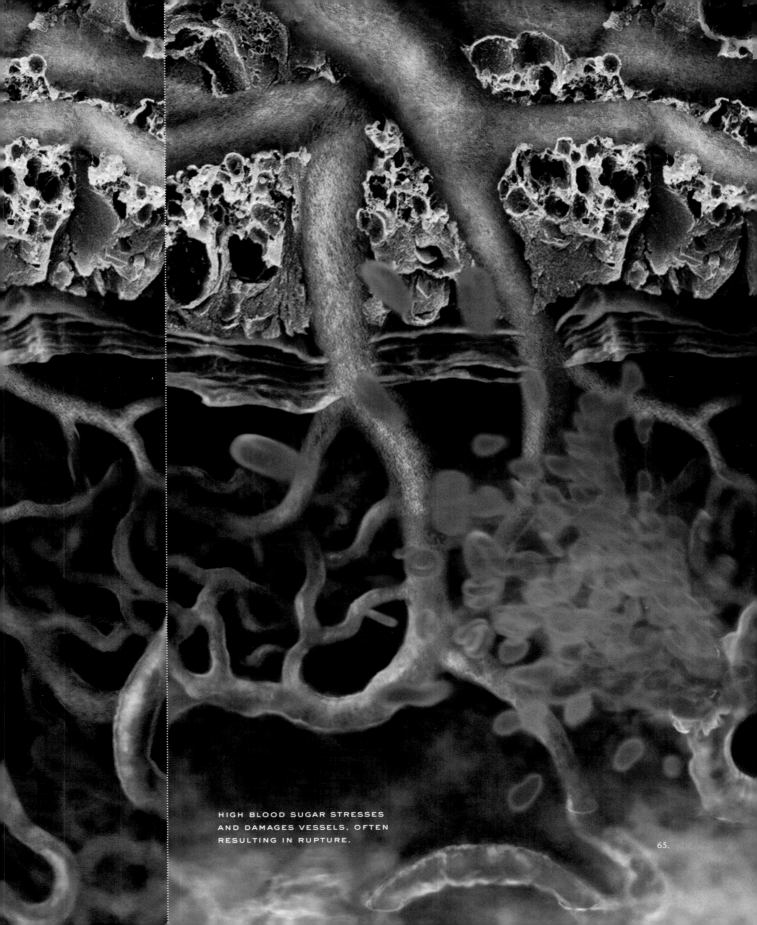

HIGH BLOOD SUGAR STRESSES
AND DAMAGES VESSELS, OFTEN
RESULTING IN RUPTURE.

65.

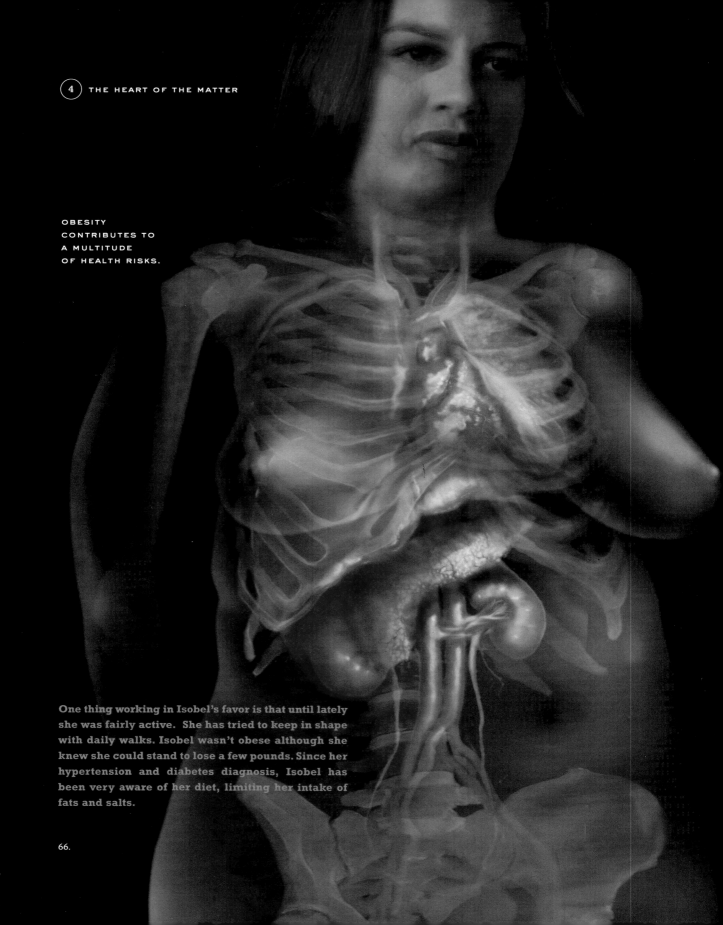

OBESITY
CONTRIBUTES TO
A MULTITUDE
OF HEALTH RISKS.

One thing working in Isobel's favor is that until lately
she was fairly active. She has tried to keep in shape
with daily walks. Isobel wasn't obese although she
knew she could stand to lose a few pounds. Since her
hypertension and diabetes diagnosis, Isobel has
been very aware of her diet, limiting her intake of
fats and salts.

66.

12	13	14	14	15	15	16	17	17	18	18	19	20	20	21	22	22	23	23	24	25	25	26
13	13	14	15	15	16	16	17	18	18	19	20	20	21	21	22	23	23	24	25	25	26	27
13	14	14	15	16	16	17	18	18	19	19	20	21	21	22	23	23	24	25	25	26	27	28
13	14	15	15	16	17	17	18	19	19	20	21	21	22	23	23	24	25	25	26	27	28	29
14	15	15	16	17	17	18	19	19	20	21	21	22	23	23	24	25	25	26	27	28	29	30
14	16	16	16	17	18	18	19	20	21	21	22	23	23	24	25	25	26	27	28	29	30	31
15	16	16	17	18	18	19	20	20	21	22	23	23	24	25	25	26	27	28	29	30	31	32
15	16	17	17	18	19	20	20	21	22	22	23	24	25	25	26	27	28	29	30	31	32	33
16	17	17	18	19	19	20	21	22	22	23	24	25	25	26	27	28	29	30	31	32	33	34
16	17	18	18	19	20	21	22	22	23	24	25	25	26	27	28	29	30	31	32	33	34	35
17	18	18	19	20	21	21	22	23	24	25	25	26	27	28	29	30	31	32	33	34	35	35
17	18	19	20	20	21	22	23	24	25	25	26	27	28	29	30	31	32	33	34	35	35	36
18	19	19	20	21	22	23	24	24	25	26	27	28	29	30	31	32	33	34	35	35	36	37
18	19	20	21	22	22	24	24	25	26	27	28	29	30	31	32	33	34	35	36	36	37	39
19	20	21	22	22	23	24	25	26	27	28	29	30	31	32	33	34	35	36	37	37	39	40
19	20	21	22	23	24	25	26	27	28	29	30	31	32	33	34	35	36	37	38	39	40	41
20	21	22	23	24	25	26	27	28	29	30	31	32	33	34	35	36	37	38	39	40	41	42
105	110	115	**120**	125	130	135	140	145	150	155	160	165	170	175	180	185	190	195	200	205	210	215

WEIGHT (LB)

< 18 Underweight   18-24 Healthy   25–29 Overweight   30–39 Obese   > 40 Morbidly Ob[ese]

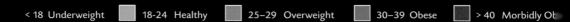

...nd its health risks are a growing problem ...ited States. It is estimated that more than ... of adults are either overweight (10 to ...s heavier than recommended) or obese ...n 30 pounds heavier than recommended)*. ...ber of overweight and obese school-age ... also on the rise. This is especially alarm- ... what is known about how obesity in- ...e risk of diabetes, high blood pressure, and ...cular disease.

...Framingham Study found that regular ...and maintaining a healthy weight are ...ctors for cardiovascular health. Your heart ...le like any other in your body. Regular exercise strengthens muscles and improves th efficiency of circulation and nutrient and wast exchange. Little or no exercise means less muscl tone and can cause weight gain, which adds stress t the cardiovascular system and increases bloo pressure. Weight gain—specifically the extra fa cells—also raises blood sugar and cholesterol levels People who are overweight or obese are at a muc higher risk of developing diabetes, which increase their risk of chronic kidney and heart disease. Peopl who are obese also take a longer time to recover fron surgical treatments and are more likely to develo complications from surgery.

*Refer to body mass index (BMI) chart

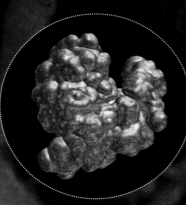

WHEN TOO MUCH LDL
CHOLESTEROL CIRCULATES
IN THE BLOOD, IT CAUSES
PLAQUE BUILDUP,
OR ATHEROSCLEROSIS.

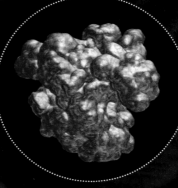

HDL CHOLESTEROL TENDS
TO CARRY PLAQUE-
BUILDING MATERIALS AWAY
FROM THE ARTERIES.

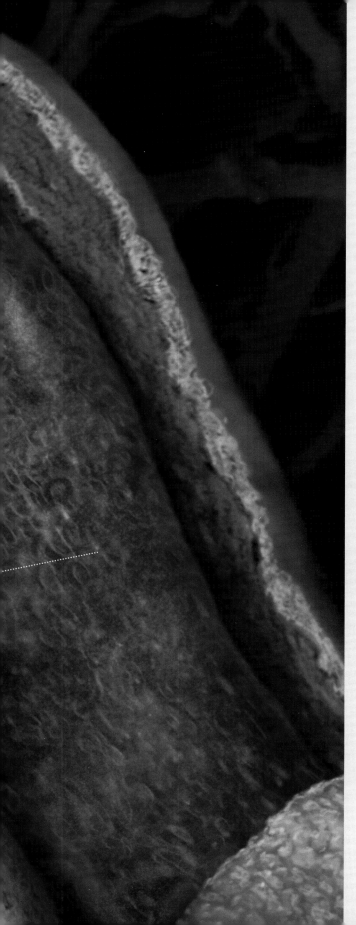

Isobel has been on medication for over ten years to treat her high blood pressure. Her doctor, Dr. Peter Fail, also recommended a diet and exercise regimen to reduce her blood cholesterol level.

Cholesterol is an important substance; it is a building block for other molecules and components of your body. Cholesterol stems from two sources: your liver, which produces cholesterol, and the foods you eat. The genes you inherit play an important role in how your body makes and metabolizes cholesterol. High cholesterol levels can run in the family and may be due to inherited conditions. However, a diet of foods high in cholesterol—meat, eggs, and dairy products—can increase the amount of cholesterol in the blood to unhealthy levels. This is often how cardiovascular problems begin. High cholesterol levels increase a person's risk of atherosclerosis and coronary heart disease. Worse, cholesterol also affects other risk factors such as hypertension, diabetes, and obesity, thus compounding the problems.

Cholesterol molecules travel through the blood attached to proteins. These packages are called lipoproteins and can be low- or high-density depending on the ratio of cholesterol to protein. Low-density lipoproteins (LDL) have more cholesterol than protein and LDL cholesterol is the biggest risk factor for heart disease. High-density lipoproteins (HDL) have more protein than cholesterol and HDL cholesterol is actually thought to protect against cardiovascular disease. HDL cholesterol may clear cholesterol from the bloodstream for disposal in the liver. Fortunately, changes in diet and/or using medication can lower cholesterol levels and reduce further disease risk. Lowering cholesterol can even reverse some of the damage that has already occurred.

CROSS-SECTIONS OF BLOOD
VESSELS REVEALING PROGRESSIVE
STAGES OF PLAQUE BUILDUP
AND ATHEROSCLEROSIS

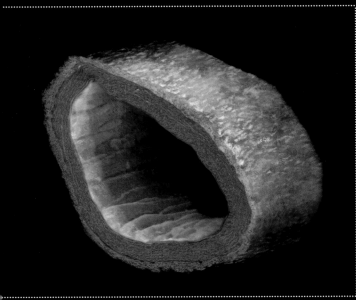

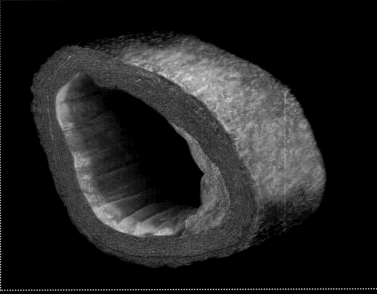

Although previously thought of as a problem of old age, the tell-tale signs of atherosclerosis—fatty streaks in the lining of the arteries—can be seen even in fetuses. High cholesterol levels in pregnant women affect the cardiovascular development of their fetuses.

Cholesterol and other fatty molecules in the blood can stick to the inner lining of arteries and be transported into the middle layer of arteries. To try to clean up the mess, the endothelial cells that make up the inner lining send out chemical signals that summon inflammatory cells. These cells invade the area and engulf the fatty molecules, leaving behind the fatty streaks. If the levels of cholesterol don't drop, the buildup continues. The fats start to accumulate faster than the cleanup process can remove them and develop into noticeable deposits known as plaque. As the plaques grow, so do the problems. The bulging plaque reduces the diameter of the arteries, which decreases blood flow and increases blood pressure. As a defense, the arteries start shoring up, making more support cells to cope with the rising blood pressure. The arteries become less flexible; hence the description of the condition as hardening of the arteries.

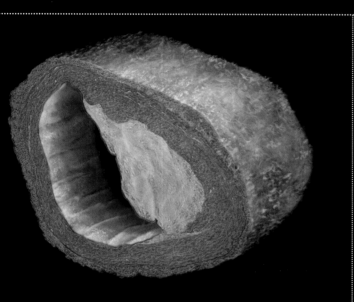

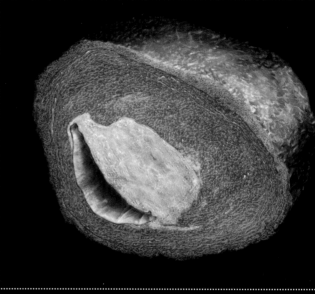

Dr. Fail is familiar with Isobel's medical history. He says: "She's definitely at risk for a heart attack. First of all, she's hypertensive. She's on medications. She's diabetic, and now she has developed angina, which she has not had before. She walks every day and all of a sudden when walking she notices chest pressure. When she stops walking, the pain goes away. This really is classic angina. Suppose we take the crystal ball approach and ask, will she have a heart attack? I have no idea, but if she came in tomorrow morning with a massive heart attack, would anybody in the room be surprised? I'd have to say no."

GUIDELINE FOR CHOLESTEROL LEVELS

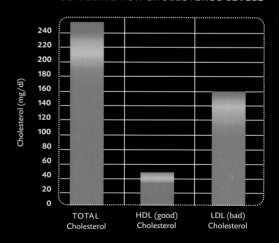

73.

Dr. Fail could tell from Isobel's ECG that her heart was not working normally. With Isobel's high blood pressure and given the suddenness of her pain, Dr. Fail worried that something might be seriously wrong. He recommended a number of tests that would measure Isobel's heart function and look at the blood flow to her heart. The results were not good: Isobel had a blockage in one of the arteries supplying her heart.

At any given time, over 6.5 million Americans are suffering from chest pains or angina. This pain may be sharp and centered in the chest or may be a dull ache that spreads to the neck, jaw, back of the shoulders or arms. Although angina is a serious condition in itself, it is also a serious warning sign that future heart trouble may be imminent.

Angina is usually the result of decreased blood flow to the muscles of the heart due to atherosclerosis and plaque buildup in the coronary arteries supplying blood to the heart. Doctors can examine the blood flow in and around the heart and visually pinpoint the blockage area by injecting an X-ray contrast dye into the patient and then taking an X-ray of the heart—this process is called an angiogram. Decreased blood flow means less oxygen and nutrients to the heart, which causes the pain. However, the biggest danger associated with atherosclerosis is that of sudden plaque rupture.

As blood pressure increases, the force of the blood flow (shear stress) can rupture the layers of

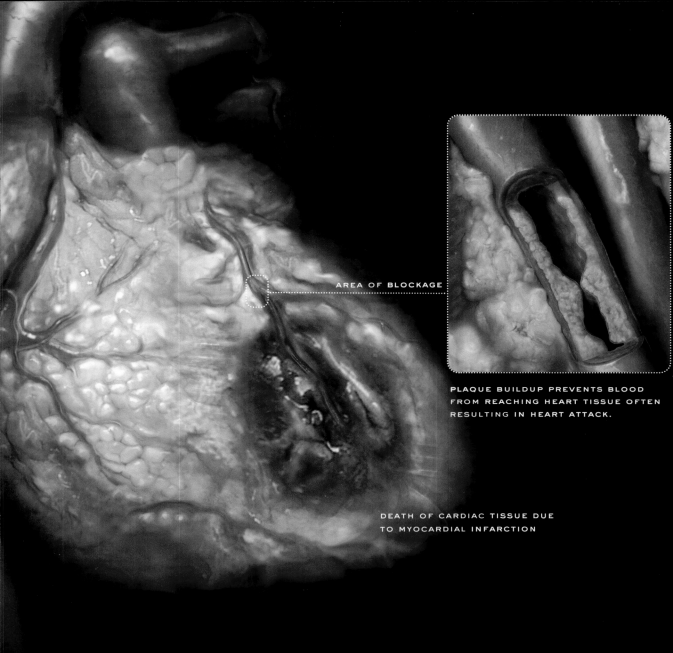

AREA OF BLOCKAGE

PLAQUE BUILDUP PREVENTS BLOOD
FROM REACHING HEART TISSUE OFTEN
RESULTING IN HEART ATTACK.

DEATH OF CARDIAC TISSUE DUE
TO MYOCARDIAL INFARCTION

cells covering the plaque and release fatty particles and other substances into the bloodstream. Your body reacts to this as it does to any injury: it starts the clotting process. Blood cells gather around the fatty particles to seal the site, which can mean that the blockage area becomes even bigger than before—large enough to block the entire vessel. Alternatively, the clot can break, be swept down the artery and get stuck downstream where the blood vessels become thinner, thereby blocking blood flow to the area.

A clot that partially or completely blocks blood flow in a coronary artery can cause the pain associated with heart attacks. These occur when the blood supply to the heart is suddenly cut off or is so drastically reduced that part of the heart stops receiving any nutrients. Heart cells begin to die. If blood supply to the heart remains cut off for four to six hours, damage to the heart is usually irreversible. Similarly, a clot in one of the arteries supplying the brain can lead to a stroke, and brain cells start to die due to lack of nutrients.

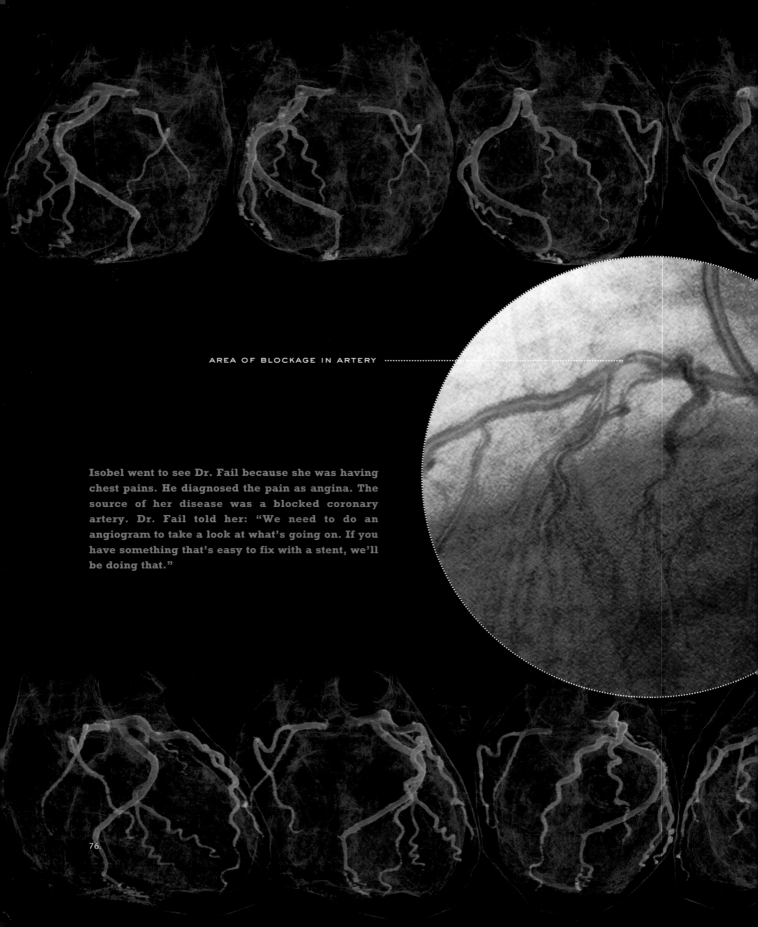

AREA OF BLOCKAGE IN ARTERY ·······································

Isobel went to see Dr. Fail because she was having chest pains. He diagnosed the pain as angina. The source of her disease was a blocked coronary artery. Dr. Fail told her: "We need to do an angiogram to take a look at what's going on. If you have something that's easy to fix with a stent, we'll be doing that."

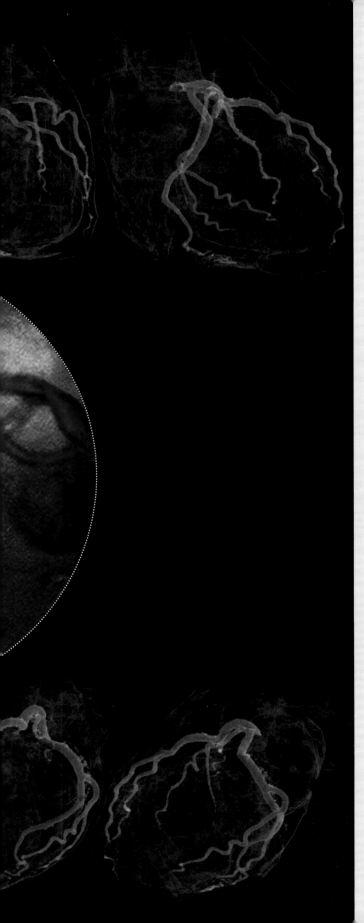

5

**how to handle a broken heart:
treating the consequences
of cardiovascular disease**

In addition to the vessels that carry blood from the
heart to the rest of the body, your heart also has its
own blood supply. The vessels that transport blood to
and from the heart are called the coronary arteries and
veins; together, they form the coronary circulation
(circulation of the heart). Your heart is one of the most
active muscles of the body, and actually receives about
5% of the blood that it circulates through the body.

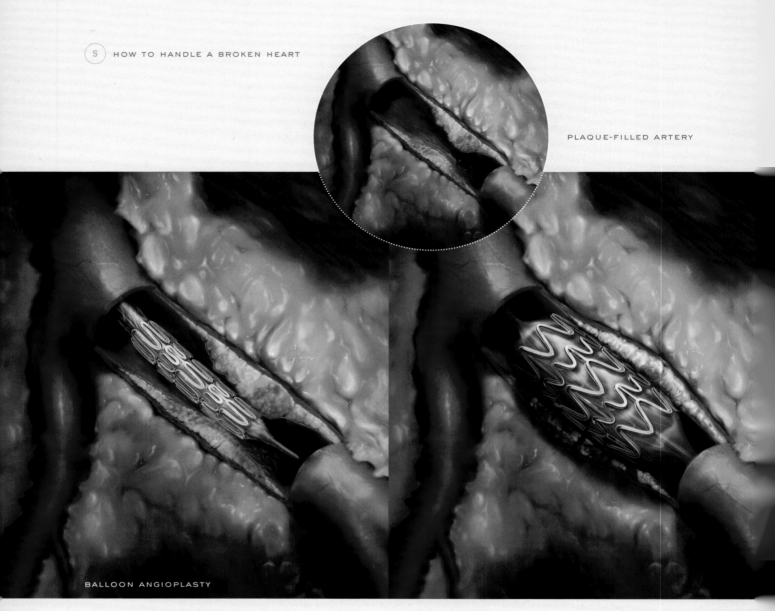

PLAQUE-FILLED ARTERY

BALLOON ANGIOPLASTY

A. A THIN STENT IS CRIMPED OVER A BALLOON
AND THREADED THROUGH THE NARROW SEGMENT
OF THE PLAQUE-FILLED ARTERY

B. PRESSURE IS USED TO INFLATE THE BALLOON,
EXPANDING THE STENT

Isobel was lucky. A balloon angioplasty cleared the artery and eased her pain. Dr. Fail acknowledged that her condition could have been a lot worse: "Isobel has been on medication for over ten years for her hypertension, and a few years ago, she started taking statins to lower her cholesterol. Without these medications, her angina could have manifested a lot earlier and be a lot more serious. She could have had a full-blown heart attack or stroke. Now we're going to continue to monitor her and adjust her medication to help her heart heal."

78.

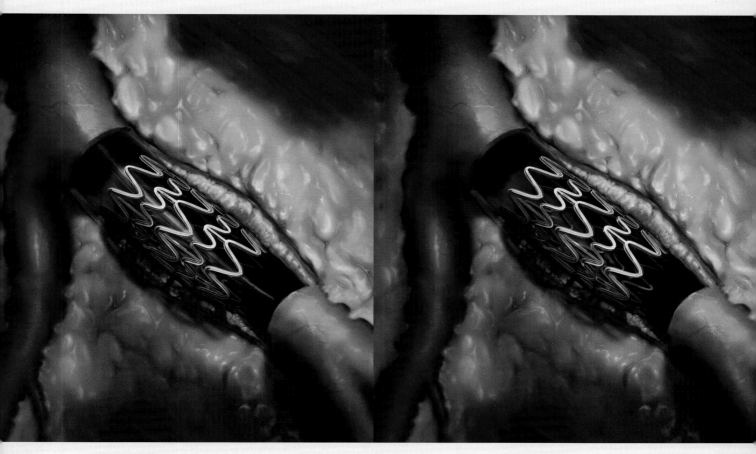

C. THE BALLOON IS DEFLATED AND REMOVED. THE STENT IS LEFT IN PLACE.

D. THE STENT PROVIDES A MECHANICAL SCAFFOLDING, WHICH PREVENTS THE COMPLETE BLOCKAGE OF THE ARTERY.

Angioplasty is the general term used for the medical procedure to open blocked arteries. There are several types of angioplasty procedures: balloon angioplasty uses a tube (catheter) with a deflated balloon located near the tip. The catheter is inserted through an artery in the arm or the groin, and threaded to the area of the blockage. The balloon is then placed across the blockage and inflated. The pressure in the balloon flattens the plaque and opens the artery. The procedure is generally done under local anesthesia and often involves a short hospital stay.

As part of the angioplasty procedure, a stent—a wire mesh netting—can be put in place to keep the artery opened. The stent may also be coated with medication to prevent clot formation and inflammation and to reduce the re-buildup of plaque.

79.

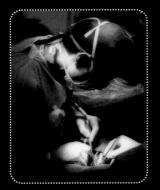

CORONARY ARTERY
BYPASS SURGERY

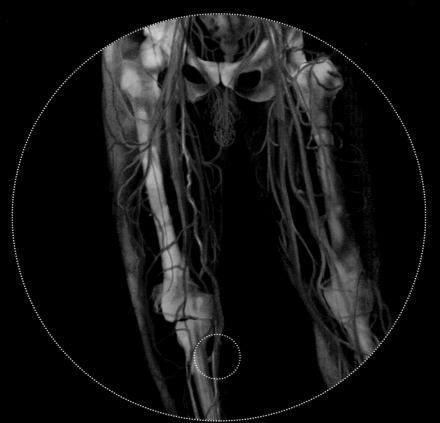

A. SECTION OF A
VEIN (GRAFT) IS TAKEN
FROM A PATIENT.

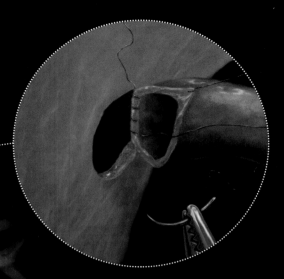

B. ONE END OF THE GRAFT IS ATTACHED TO AN ARTERY ABOVE THE BLOCKAGE.

C. THE OTHER END OF THE GRAFT IS ATTACHED TO THE CORONARY ARTERY BELOW THE BLOCKAGE.

If blockages are too widespread to be repaired by angioplasty, patients may be candidates for coronary artery bypass surgery. During bypass surgery, a section of an artery or vein from a different part of the body (usually from the leg) is removed and used to bypass the blockage (A-C). This provides a new route for blood flow.

If blood flow to the heart is reduced to the point that it causes angina, restoring blood flow or reducing the work that the heart has to do becomes extremely important. Left untreated, the reduced blood flow that causes angina can lead to a heart attack. When the blood supply to the heart is suddenly cut off or drastically reduced, even for a few minutes, heart cells begin to die, sometimes causing damage that can lead to permanent disability or death.

Today, thanks to advances in medical treatment, many people survive their heart attacks. However, heart attacks do cause irreversible damage and the extent of this damage depends on the size of the affected area and the length of time the heart muscle in the area was deprived of blood. These damaged areas or walls of the heart can prevent the heart from working properly, leading to heart failure.

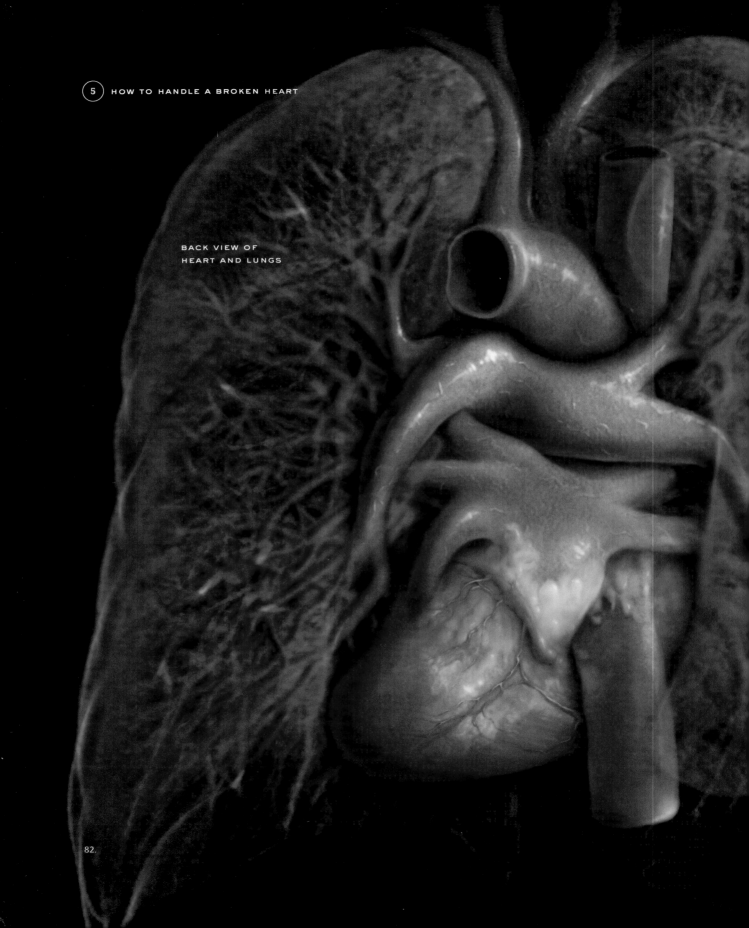

BACK VIEW OF
HEART AND LUNGS

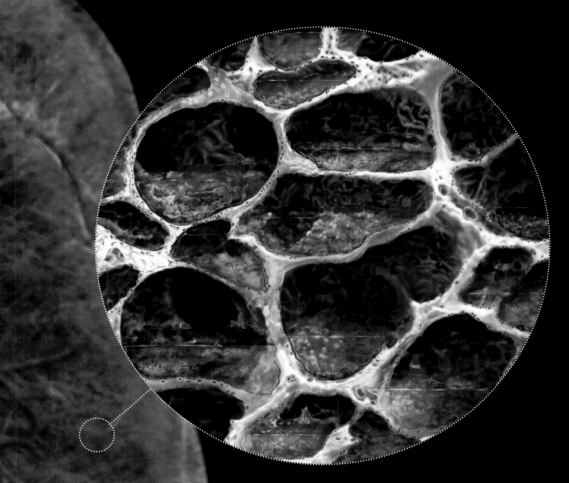

FLUID-FILLED ALVEOLI WITHIN THE LUNGS

Congestive heart failure is a condition that is becoming more common as better treatments and improved lifestyle changes ensure higher heart attack and cardiovascular disease survival. Patients diagnosed with heart failure have hearts that are not working properly. The heart cannot pump blood efficiently and blood returning to the heart sometimes backs up and causes fluid to leak from the veins and capillaries into body tissues. Different parts of the body like the legs can swell (pedal edema). A more serious condition occurs when fluid collects in the lungs (pulmonary edema) and interferes with breathing.

Medications that ease the amount of work the heart has to do can help patients who have heart failure. Nitroglycerin is often prescribed to be taken when someone is having an angina episode—it works quickly to dilate the blood vessels and increase blood flow to the heart.

83.

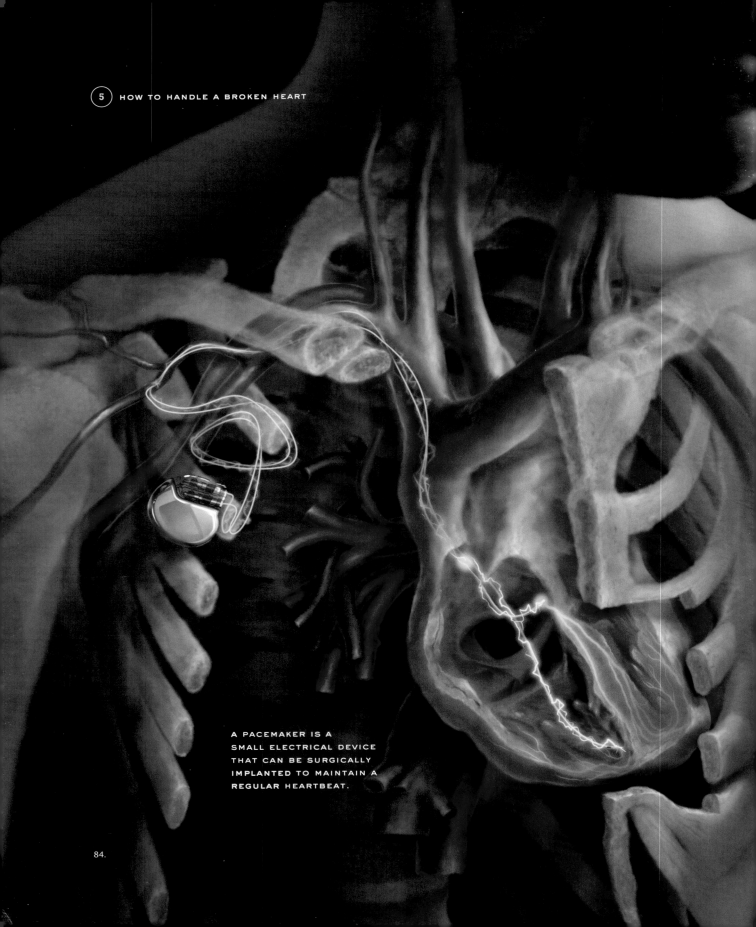

A PACEMAKER IS A
SMALL ELECTRICAL DEVICE
THAT CAN BE SURGICALLY
IMPLANTED TO MAINTAIN A
REGULAR HEARTBEAT.

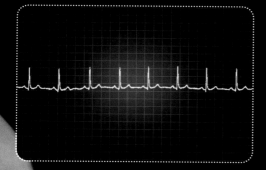

ECG: NORMAL HEARTBEAT

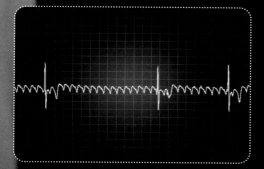

ECG: ABNORMAL HEARTBEAT

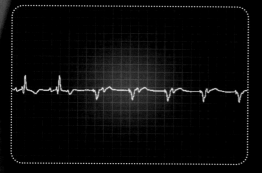

ECG: ABNORMAL HEARTBEAT
BEING CHARGED BY PACEMAKER

Patients with heart failure resulting from a heart attack usually have an enlarged heart. This occurs as the result of what is known as remodeling or changes to the heart due to muscle damage and scar tissue. Another complication of a heart attack is arrhythmia—in which the electrical activity of the heart goes haywire.

Scar tissue formed as a result of damage cannot conduct the electrical signals of the heart from one cell to another, and as a result a patient may experience irregular heartbeats or skipped beats. A specific type of arrhythmia—ventricular arrhythmia—can cause sudden cardiac death and is thought to be responsible for half of all deaths due to heart disease in the United States. Occasionally, a defect in the heart's electrical system can cause the heart to beat at a very slow rate. This condition is generally treated with a pacemaker.

A pacemaker is a small electrical device that can be surgically implanted to help maintain a regular heartbeat. Pacemakers send electrical signals to stimulate the heart to beat in proper rhythm. They can be programmed to meet the electrical needs of the heart and are now so advanced they can even be programmed to increase heartbeat with exercise and slow the heartbeat once the exercise period is over.

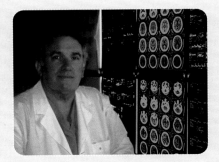

When a patient makes an appointment to see James Goodreau, M.D., it's because they've heard what an excellent doctor he is. And it's true, Dr. Goodreau is articulate, skilled, and respected by patients and colleagues alike. He is the co-director of the vascular laboratory at Lehigh Valley Hospital (Muhlenberg) in Allentown, Pennsylvania. His training has given him an excellent understanding of cardiovascular health, and his surgical skills have helped save many lives. Dr. Goodreau also has a window into his patients' lives that makes him particularly able to empathize with their experience, because in 1998 Dr. Goodreau, like many of his patients was the victim of a stroke.

The heart is not the only organ that can be affected by cardiovascular disease. Ischemic strokes happen when blockage occurs in the arteries leading to, and within, the brain. Strokes cause brain damage, which can lead to paralysis and/or loss of language, motor control, or vision, as well as other problems.

A blocked artery in the brain may be caused by a blood clot or advanced atherosclerosis. If the layers of cells covering a plaque are ruptured, a clot may form around the site to try and seal in the fatty particles. A person suffers a thrombotic stroke if a clot forms in the artery and blocks blood flow to the brain. An embolic stroke happens when a clot breaks off from its original site and moves through the bloodstream to block one of the smaller arteries in the brain. In both cases, blood supply is cut off to the affected part of the brain, and within minutes the brain cells start to die.

Embolic strokes tend to occur very suddenly. In contrast, thrombotic strokes may occur slowly over a period of time, and may actually be preceded by transient ischemic attacks (TIAs). TIAs, or mini-strokes, occur when the blood supply to an area of the brain is cut off, or vastly decreased, for a short period of time. TIAs and thrombotic strokes usually occur in people with high cholesterol levels and atherosclerosis.

Blood thinners and clot busters are medications for people at high risk of developing clots or who have developed a clot. Blood thinners do not actually thin blood; they decrease the ability of your blood to form clots. They may be prescribed for patients with high cholesterol levels and atherosclerosis to reduce the risk of strokes and heart attacks. Clot busters dissolve already-formed clots, which may be causing the stroke or heart attack.

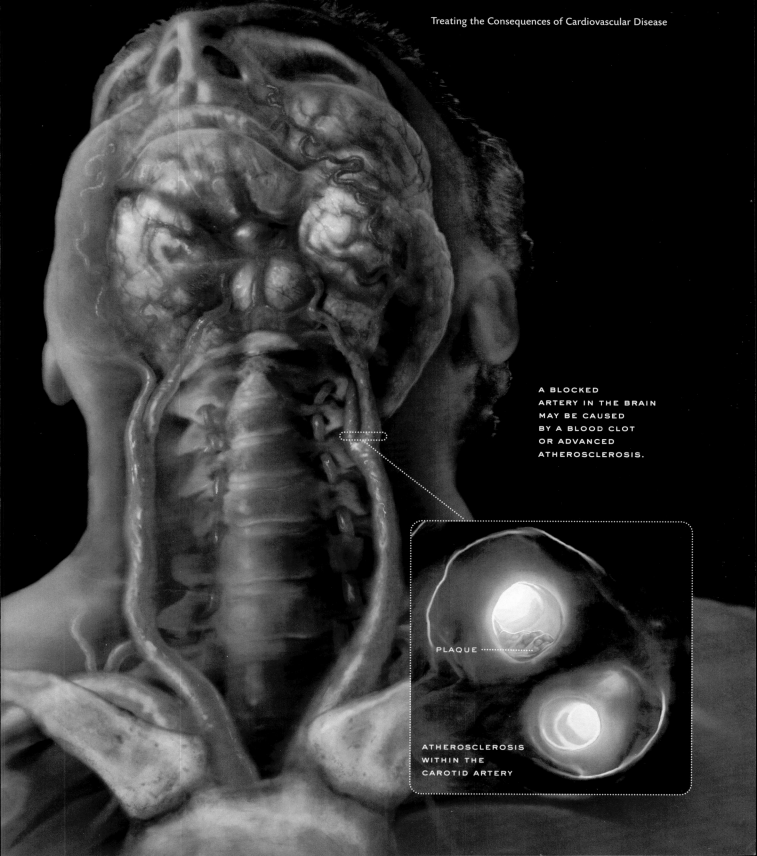

A BLOCKED
ARTERY IN THE BRAIN
MAY BE CAUSED
BY A BLOOD CLOT
OR ADVANCED
ATHEROSCLEROSIS.

PLAQUE

ATHEROSCLEROSIS
WITHIN THE
CAROTID ARTERY

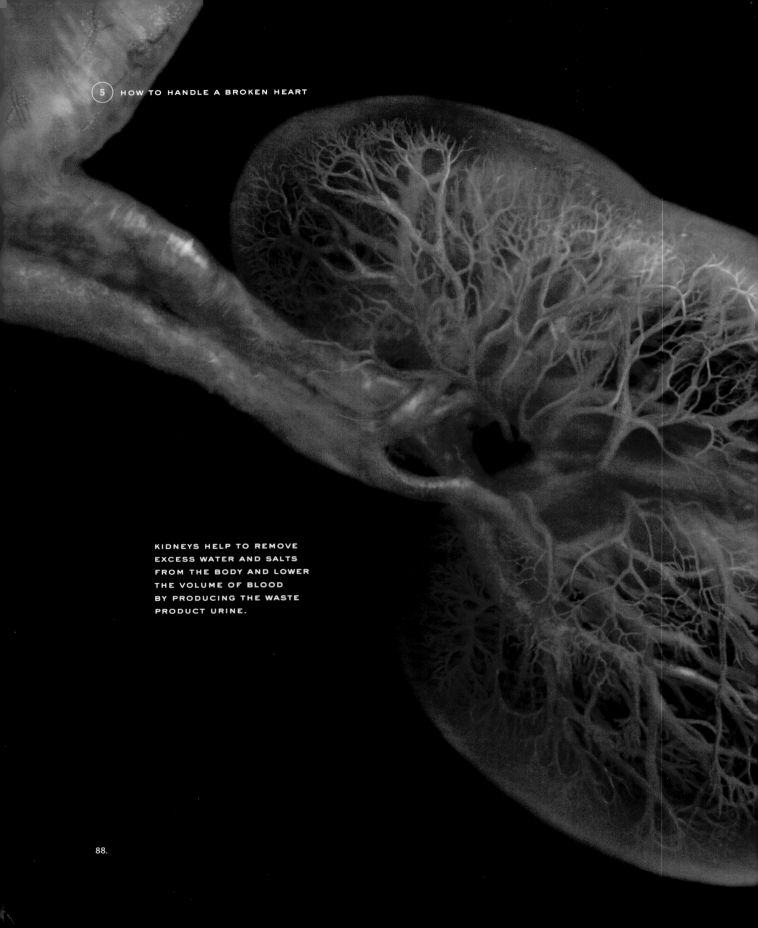

KIDNEYS HELP TO REMOVE
EXCESS WATER AND SALTS
FROM THE BODY AND LOWER
THE VOLUME OF BLOOD
BY PRODUCING THE WASTE
PRODUCT URINE.

There are four types of medication used to treat high blood pressure. Each type works on a different mechanism of blood pressure regulation.

Diuretics cause the kidneys to remove excess water and salts from the body and lower the volume of blood. Beta-blockers slow down the action of the heart by blocking the action of the chemical messenger noradrenaline. The heart doesn't work as hard to pump blood through the vessels, thus allowing blood pressure to drop. Beta-blockers are also prescribed for patients with angina and arrhythmia to help ease the symptoms of these disorders. Calcium channel blockers prevent calcium from entering the muscle cells in the walls of blood vessels. This helps keep the muscles relaxed and the blood vessels more flexible.

Angiotensin receptor blockers (ARBs) and angiotensin converting enzyme (ACE) inhibitors both work by interfering with the actions of angiotensin II—a molecule used by your body to control vessel contraction and thus blood pressure. ARBs block the action of angiotensin II and relax blood vessels. ACE inhibitors decrease the production of angiotensin II in the body. With less angiotensin II, the blood vessels are more relaxed and blood pressure decreases.

Hypertension causes damage with every heartbeat. By lowering blood pressure to the appropriate level, the damage can be minimized and potentially stopped. Most patients will require more than one medication to get their blood pressure down to healthy levels.

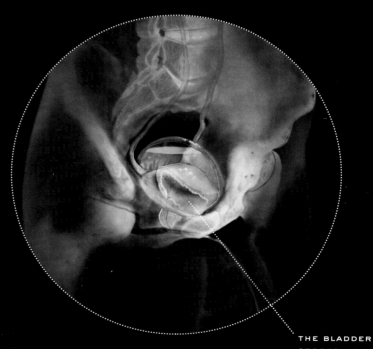

THE BLADDER
STORES URINE
UNTIL IT IS
RELEASED FROM
THE BODY.

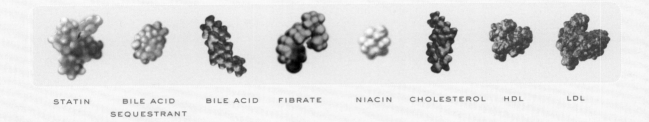

STATIN   BILE ACID   BILE ACID   FIBRATE   NIACIN   CHOLESTEROL   HDL   LDL
          SEQUESTRANT

Patients often have multiple diseases and therefore take multiple medications. It is not unusual to see patients taking medications for hypertension, heart failure, diabetes, and high cholesterol. High cholesterol may cause plaque buildup and put you at risk for atherosclerosis. Although changes in diet can lower cholesterol levels and reduce fat intake, sometimes medication is necessary. Statins, fibrates, niacin, and bile acid sequestrants are the four main types of cholesterol-reducing medications.

Statins work by blocking the action of the molecule that controls cholesterol production in the body. Statins also increase your liver's ability to remove LDL cholesterol already in the bloodstream (A). For most patients, statins are the most effective cholesterol reduction medication with the least side effects.

Fibrates and niacin increase the level of HDL cholesterol, which then lowers LDL levels (B). Fibrates also increase the breakdown of triglycerides; this is the chemical form in which most fats exist in food and in your body. People with high cholesterol levels usually have high triglyceride levels. High triglyceride levels in the blood have also been linked to coronary heart disease and diabetes.

Bile acid sequestrants bind and eliminate bile acids from the body (C). Bile acids are produced in the liver from cholesterol, and help with the absorption of dietary fats and cholesterol. The net effect of bile acid sequestrants as medication is to increase bile acid production and decrease cholesterol levels in the blood.

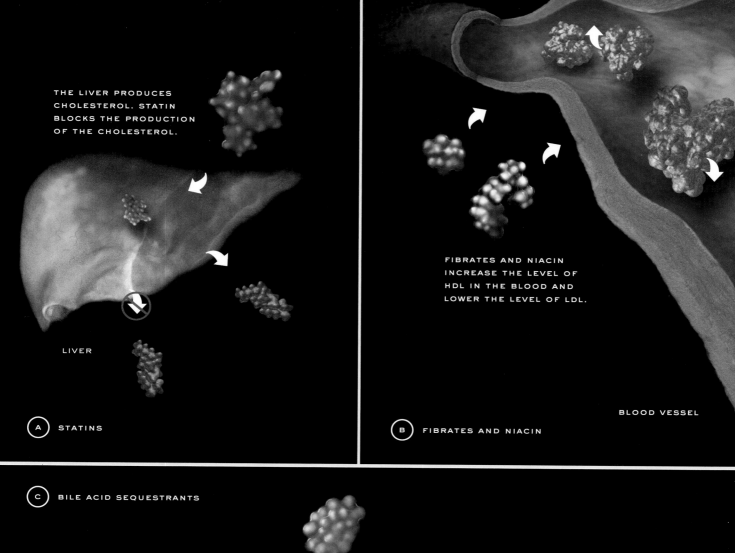

THE LIVER PRODUCES
CHOLESTEROL. STATIN
BLOCKS THE PRODUCTION
OF THE CHOLESTEROL.

LIVER

(A) STATINS

FIBRATES AND NIACIN
INCREASE THE LEVEL OF
HDL IN THE BLOOD AND
LOWER THE LEVEL OF LDL.

BLOOD VESSEL

(B) FIBRATES AND NIACIN

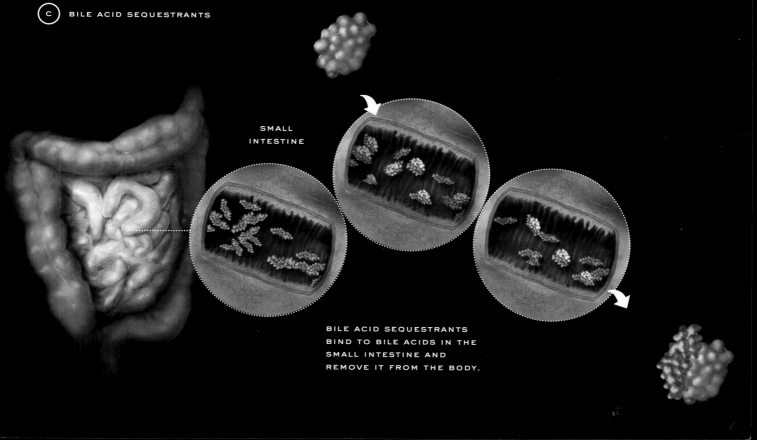

(C) BILE ACID SEQUESTRANTS

SMALL
INTESTINE

BILE ACID SEQUESTRANTS
BIND TO BILE ACIDS IN THE
SMALL INTESTINE AND
REMOVE IT FROM THE BODY.

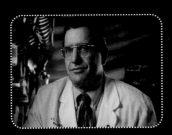

The culprits, or the biological terrorists, in heart disease are well known and easily identified. John Castaldo, M.D., chief of neurology at Lehigh Valley Hospital in Allentown, Pennsylvania, says: "They are high blood pressure; they are diabetes; they are smoking; they are high cholesterol. They are almost always possible to treat and easy to avoid."

As both Drs. Castaldo and Goodreau know, having the ability to defeat the enemies of cardiovascular health doesn't necessarily mean being able to eradicate the problems. Says Dr. Castaldo: "In this country, 70% of the hypertensive population is not treated adequately, and less than a third of people with high cholesterol are on any treatment at all. More importantly, if you have high blood pressure and you have high cholesterol, those two things together increase your risk more than one plus one." High blood pressure and high cholesterol, in other words, make each other worse. They work together in horrible synergy to more quickly damage a person's body.

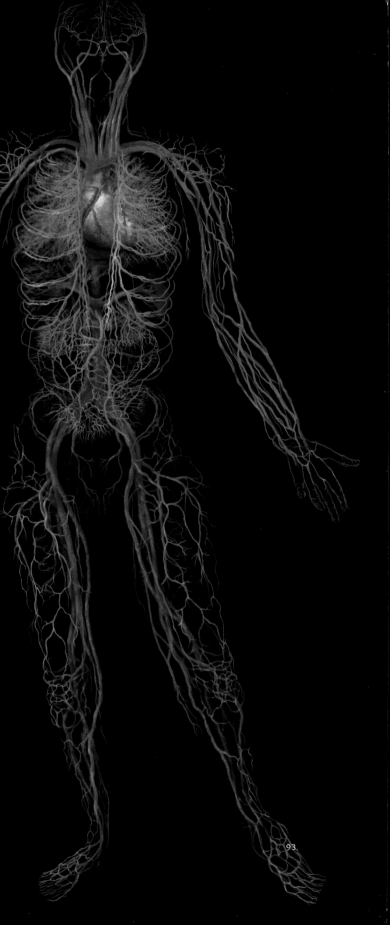

People with cardiovascular problems may need to take a number of different types of medications. They may also need medication for other complications such as diabetes and chronic kidney disease. Medications work best if patients take them as prescribed by their health-care professional. Unfortunately, drug compliance—taking medication regularly as directed—especially for those with hypertension, is a growing problem.

Half of all hypertensive patients are not taking their medication regularly. In the short term, people with hypertension may not feel any symptoms and the medication, which can cause side effects, frequently seems more unpleasant than the disease.

However, for the long term, treatment is essential for a person with hypertension to live a longer and healthier life.

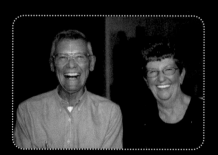

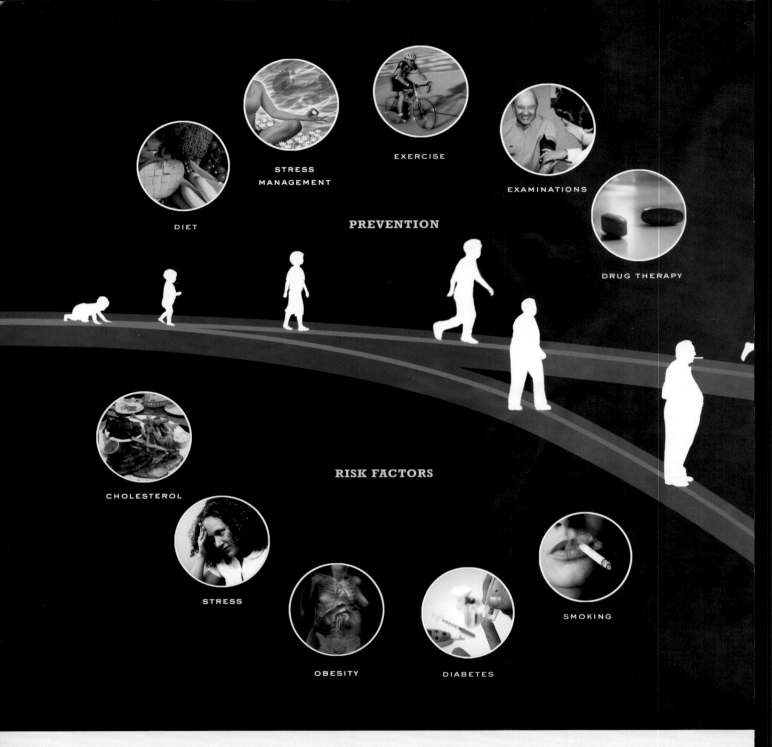

DIET

STRESS
MANAGEMENT

EXERCISE

EXAMINATIONS

PREVENTION

DRUG THERAPY

CHOLESTEROL

RISK FACTORS

STRESS

SMOKING

OBESITY

DIABETES

From conception to birth and throughout your life, many factors affect your cardiovascular health. Studies such as the Framingham Heart Study continue to identify factors—genetic, behavioral, and environmental—that change and remodel the cardiovascular system. This ongoing process of change and remodeling of the cardiovascular system is referred to as the cardiovascular continuum.

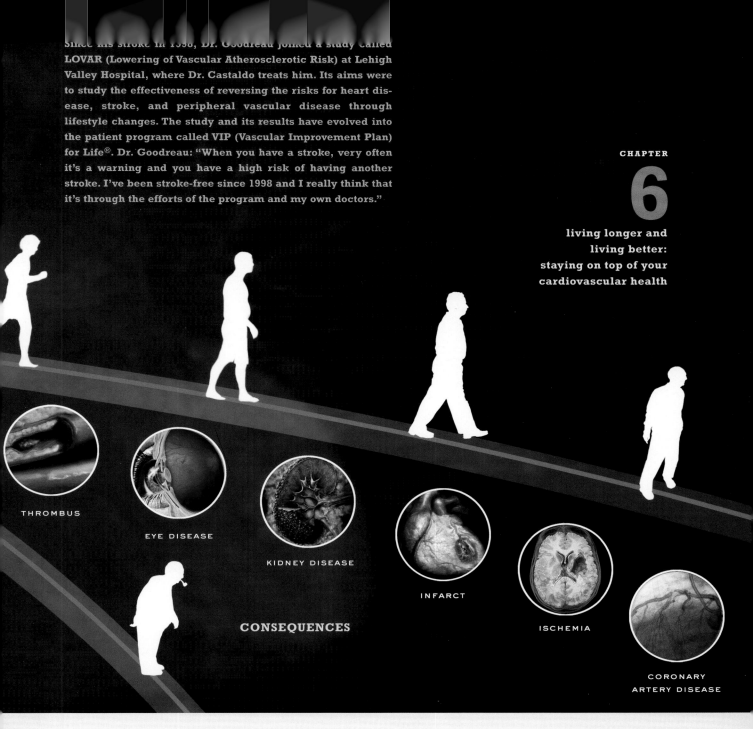

Since his stroke in 1998, Dr. Goodreau joined a study called LOVAR (Lowering of Vascular Atherosclerotic Risk) at Lehigh Valley Hospital, where Dr. Castaldo treats him. Its aims were to study the effectiveness of reversing the risks for heart disease, stroke, and peripheral vascular disease through lifestyle changes. The study and its results have evolved into the patient program called VIP (Vascular Improvement Plan) for Life®. Dr. Goodreau: "When you have a stroke, very often it's a warning and you have a high risk of having another stroke. I've been stroke-free since 1998 and I really think that it's through the efforts of the program and my own doctors."

CHAPTER

6

living longer and
living better:
staying on top of your
cardiovascular health

THROMBUS

EYE DISEASE

KIDNEY DISEASE

INFARCT

ISCHEMIA

CORONARY
ARTERY DISEASE

CONSEQUENCES

You move along the cardiovascular continuum at various speeds depending on your risk factors. A person's genetic makeup affects where they start on the continuum. Eating a high-fat diet can speed a person along the continuum, as can stress and hypertension. All of this is not to say that these changes are inevitable. Avoiding or delaying both atherosclerosis and hypertension is possible for most people with appropriate diet, exercise, and medical care, but most people will progress along the cardiovascular continuum to some degree before they die.

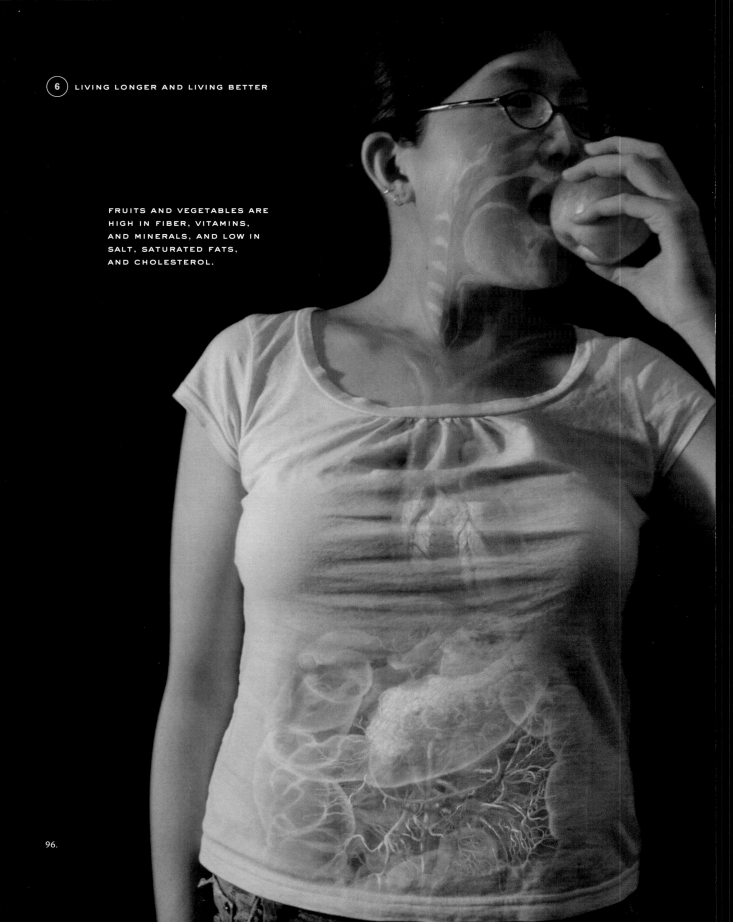

FRUITS AND VEGETABLES ARE
HIGH IN FIBER, VITAMINS,
AND MINERALS, AND LOW IN
SALT, SATURATED FATS,
AND CHOLESTEROL.

A healthy diet is a useful and effective tool in preventing cardiovascular damage and slowing your progress along the cardiovascular continuum. Healthy eating should focus on reducing the three main risk factors: high salt, which can lead to hypertension; high blood cholesterol, which can lead to atherosclerosis; and high caloric content, which can lead to excess weight and further stress on the cardiovascular system.

Start by reviewing all the foods you regularly consume during the course of a week, and rate the items for their nutritional value. By doing so, you can make decisions about how best to change and improve your diet. In general, processed and fast foods are poor choices as they are high in salt, calories, triglycerides, and saturated fats—a form of fat that is usually solid at room temperature. All animal fats are saturated and can increase blood cholesterol levels.

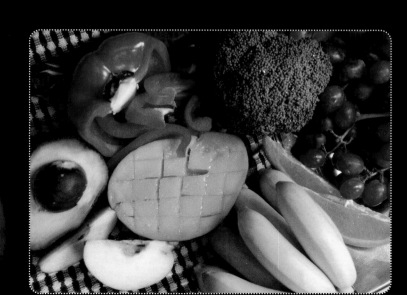

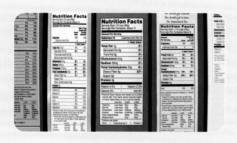

It is always a good idea to read the packaging labels and be more aware of your choices; most brands offer low-salt, low-sugar, and/or additive-free options. Alternatively, use fresh ingredients and prepare the food yourself so that you can control the portion size and the nutritional content. Instead of getting protein from red meat, which is high in cholesterol and saturated fats, consider substituting poultry, legumes, soy products, or fish. Fish such as trout, salmon, and tuna are high in omega-3 fatty acids, which make blood less likely to clot, thus lowering the risk of heart attacks and other cardiovascular problems. Omega-3 fatty acids also lower blood pressure and triglyceride levels, and increase good HDL cholesterol levels.

Both the American Heart Association and the U.S. Department of Agriculture (USDA) recommend daily portions of fruits and vegetables, which are high in fiber, vitamins, and minerals, and low in salt, saturated fats, and cholesterol. Green, leafy vegetables such as spinach and broccoli are high in folic acid and vitamin B, which control the levels of an amino acid—homocysteine—in the blood. Homocysteine can cause nicks in the arterial wall and promote the development of atherosclerosis.

Diet and nutrition are some of the main lifestyle issues that programs like LOVAR and VIP for Life® try to address. Research has already identified the heart-healthy quality of certain diets. Dr. Castaldo says, "We know that people in cultures that eat a lot of fish, fresh fruits, and vegetables can live a long life without any signs of atherosclerosis. We also know that when these same cultures migrate to the United States and switch to a U.S. fast food diet high in cholesterol and low in fresh fruits and vegetables, they develop the same types of cardiovascular disease that Americans get. So, a big factor in cardiovascular disease risk is clearly what we're eating. We're not getting enough fresh fruits and vegetables, and we're eating too much in the way of high-fat foods."

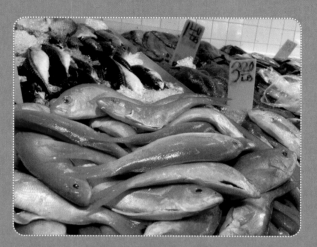

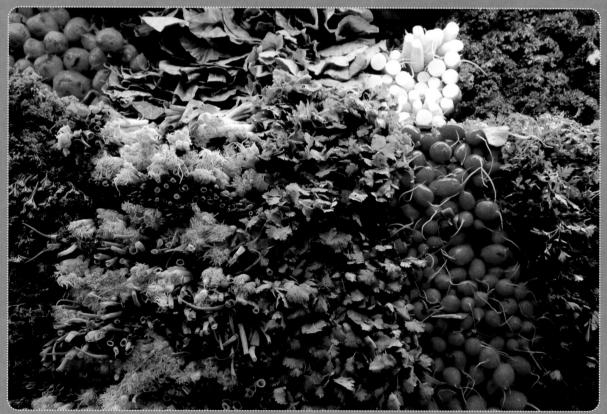

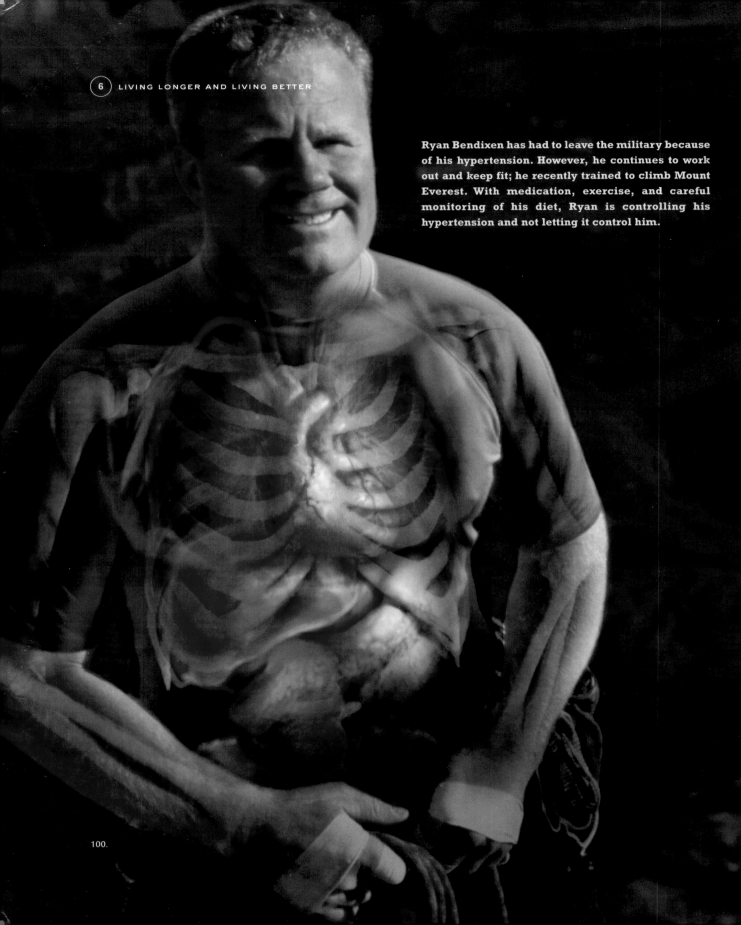

Ryan Bendixen has had to leave the military because of his hypertension. However, he continues to work out and keep fit; he recently trained to climb Mount Everest. With medication, exercise, and careful monitoring of his diet, Ryan is controlling his hypertension and not letting it control him.

Dr. Goodreau has learned to be more careful about his diet and his lifestyle choices. "The lessons I've learned from my own experience I translate to my patients. Before my stroke, I was overweight, my cholesterol was up. I wasn't smoking, but I wasn't doing anything in terms of exercise other than working." Dr. Goodreau continues to follow the advice from the original LOVAR program—the preservation of cardiovascular health is a lifelong commitment.

Maintaining a healthy weight is one of the foundations for the preservation of cardiovascular health. For those who have exceeded their recommended weight (refer to BMI chart on p. 67), the best way to lose weight is to reduce caloric intake and increase physical activity. A moderately-active person needs about 15 calories to maintain one pound per day; someone who is 150 pounds needs a caloric intake of 2,250 per day to keep his or her weight at 150 pounds. In order to lose weight, you need to reduce the caloric intake and/or use up calories through physical activity. Reducing your intake by 500 calories per day can mean a weight loss of one to two pounds a week, which is the recommended rate as it reflects weight loss from fat as opposed to muscle mass or water loss. Slow and steady weight loss also helps you and your body adjust to changes in diet and physical activity levels.

Regular physical activity helps to maintain fitness levels, which directly reduces the risk of disease and death. Even individuals with preexisting heart conditions are frequently prescribed mild exercise regimens by their healthcare professional in order to keep their health from deteriorating further. If you are overweight or have a medical condition, speak to your healthcare professional about how best to begin an exercise program. If you have not been physically active, it is a good idea to start slowly with moderate physical activity like walking, and gradually build up to the American Heart Association and the USDA-recommended 30 minutes of physical activity a day.

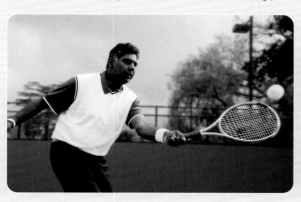

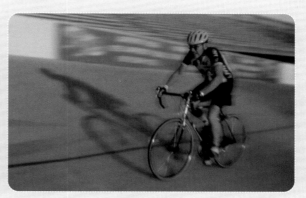

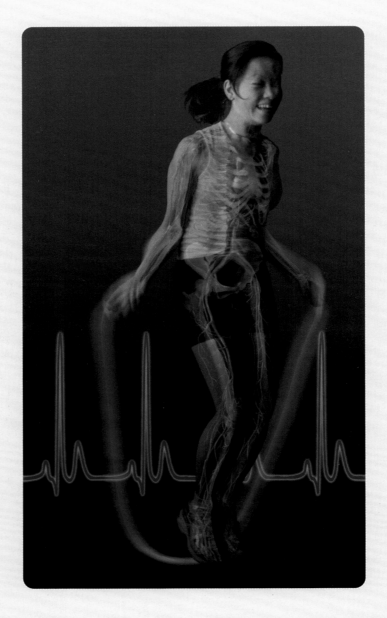

Quality is as important as quantity—most people want to live long and live well. Dr. Castaldo says, "I know people who were ravaged by heart attack, who had pain in their legs when they walked—a clear warning sign of vascular disease. These people are now riding their bicycles in the velodrome, jogging every day, playing golf, and doing things they never dreamed that they could do. They have taken the risk factors to heart and they have changed their lives. Education can work."

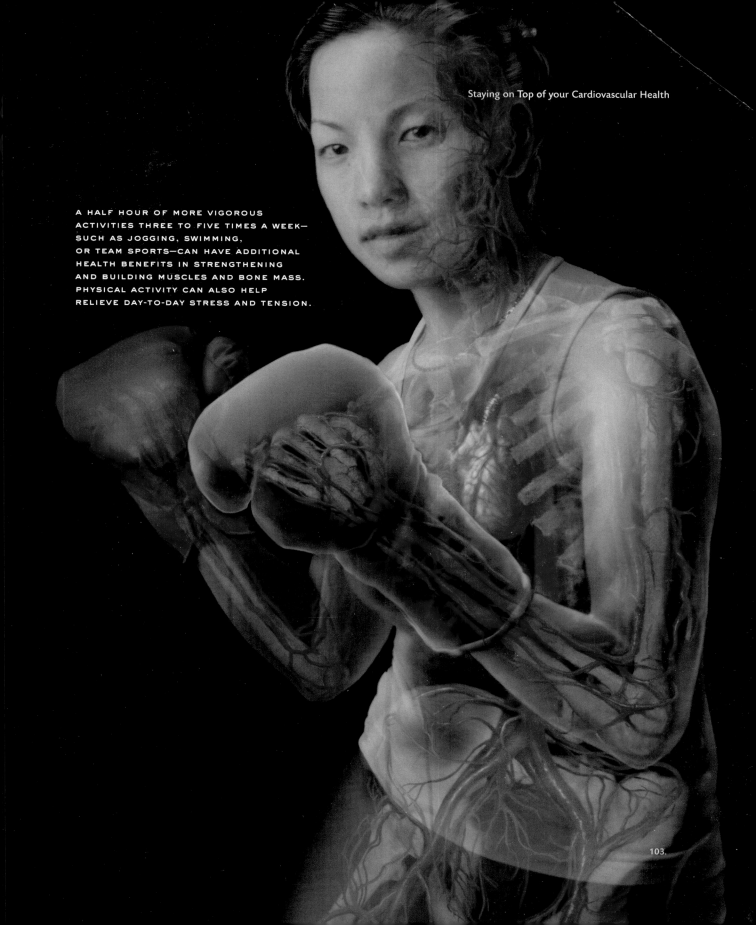

A HALF HOUR OF MORE VIGOROUS
ACTIVITIES THREE TO FIVE TIMES A WEEK—
SUCH AS JOGGING, SWIMMING,
OR TEAM SPORTS—CAN HAVE ADDITIONAL
HEALTH BENEFITS IN STRENGTHENING
AND BUILDING MUSCLES AND BONE MASS.
PHYSICAL ACTIVITY CAN ALSO HELP
RELIEVE DAY-TO-DAY STRESS AND TENSION.

Dr. Castaldo believes that healthcare costs can be reduced if there is more of a focus on prevention. "We as a nation are so enamored with high tech. We love bypasses, angioplasties, stents, and clot retrievers. We think this is what treating cardio-vascular disease is all about. And yet, the real important mission of healthcare professionals in this country and for patients too is to treat the under-lying causes of the disease from as early an age as possible. Every year, we spend $300 billion for the care of patients with cardiovascular disease. I think we can do better by putting more of that money toward prevention, treating the blood pressure, treating the diabetes, creating programs for stopping smoking, and educating the public about the importance of maintaining and preserving cardiovascular health."

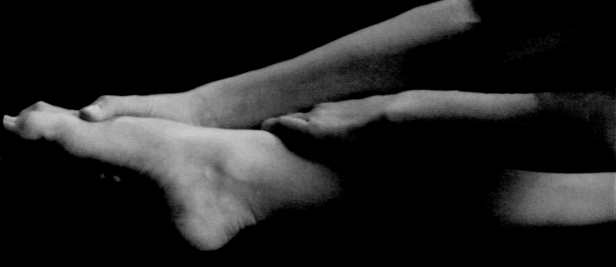

Stress, or more accurately poor stress management, can have detrimental effects on your overall health. Under stressful conditions, your body's hormonal glands release adrenaline to prepare for a physical response known as fight or flight. Adrenaline increases heart rate, blood pressure, and blood sugar to provide the body with an energy surge, which can disrupt your body's ability to relax after the stressful conditions are over. The down time afterwards is also when you become more prone to infections—components of adrenaline and other stress-related hormones suppress the immune system. Research shows that chronic mental stress causes the inner layers of blood vessels to con-tract and can decrease blood flow to the heart and brain

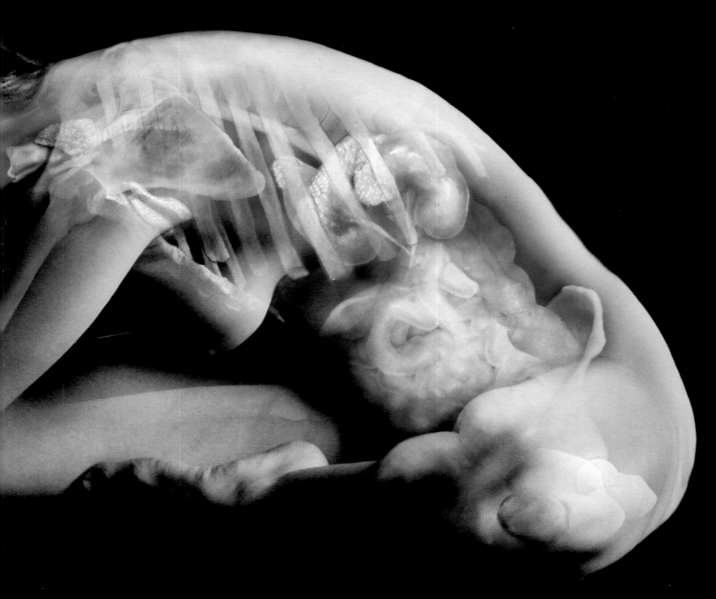

and increase the risk of heart attacks and strokes. Humor, relaxation, and exercise have the opposite effect on the risk of heart attacks and strokes.

Physical activity can help relieve stress as can meditation or yoga. The stretches and poses in yoga can increase joint flexibility and help with breathing and posture. Yoga is also a good way to build strength and bone density—worked muscles stimulate bone buildup and decrease the risk for osteoporosis while burning calories. Different activities work for different people as stress relief—the important thing is to be able to recognize the signs of stress and find ways to deal with it in a positive way.

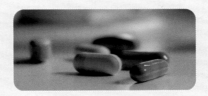

A different type of stress—oxidative stress—is a natural process that occurs in your body. As a part of the metabolic process, free radicals—atoms or a group of atoms with unpaired electrons—can be formed when oxygen interacts with certain molecules. Free radicals are also created when your body is exposed to pollution, radiation, or cigarette smoke. Normally, your body uses antioxidants to mop up and eliminate free radicals before they can react with and damage cells and DNA. Free radical damage has been linked to arterial aging and cancer. Vitamin C and vitamin E are excellent antioxidants and can be obtained from a healthy diet high in fruits and vegetables. A well-balanced diet should supply enough of these and other necessary vitamins (A, B, D), and minerals (zinc, iron, potassium, selenium). However, taking a daily multivitamin supplement is recommended as a safety net and to guard against long-term damage.

Supplements should never be considered a replacement source of vitamins and minerals, which tend to work best when absorbed from food.

In addition to a multivitamin, research suggests that a daily baby dose of aspirin (half of an adult pill or 162 milligrams) may have a beneficial effect for those at risk of cardiovascular disease. The active ingredient in aspirin—acetylsalicylic acid—has long been used as a medication to relieve pain and inflammation. Aspirin also slows down clot production, which can lead to a heart attack or stroke.

Consult a healthcare professional as to the recommended daily dose of vitamins and supplements that work best for you. Aspirin can cause stomach upset and too much of any one vitamin can be harmful to your health. Some vitamins can interfere with prescribed medication, especially statins.

A FREE RADICAL IS FORMED WHEN A CHEMICAL REACTION
BREAKS THE BONDS THAT HOLD A MOLECULE'S PAIRED
ELECTRONS TOGETHER. A FREE RADICAL CONTAINS AN
ODD NUMBER OF ELECTRONS, MAKING IT VERY UNSTABLE,
REACTIVE, AND DAMAGING TO THE BODY.

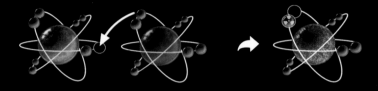

FREE RADICAL

ENVIRONMENTAL FACTORS MAY RESULT IN THE
INCREASE OF FREE RADICALS IN YOUR BODY.

A HEALTHY DIET CAN HELP REDUCE THE
NUMBER OF FREE RADICALS IN YOUR BODY.

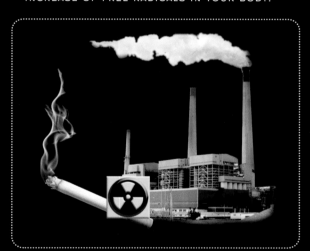

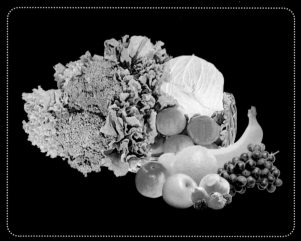

Programs like LOVAR and VIP for Life ® have professionals who can recommend diet and exercise regimens along with stress management, smoking cessation, and diabetes management. They also help patients monitor and track their progress through diagnostic tests and checkups in conjunction with their primary care physician. It is still up to the patient to follow through and keep up the lifestyle changes. Says Dr. Goodreau: "We have a disease that is out of control and somewhere along the way we have to prevent the disease, not just treat it. Programs like LOVAR should be developed across the country. The old saying 'an ounce of prevention is worth a pound of cure' is for real."

Regular medical checkups are essential for achieving positive outcomes. A person with high cholesterol levels and hypertension may not have any symptoms until stricken by the heart attack or stroke. Without information and education, it is nearly impossible to initiate and maintain lifestyle changes or the treatments needed to improve cardiovascular health. Reversing a lifetime of damage can take a lot of work.

Once successful changes are made, they need to be maintained. A healthy diet and regular physical activity should be part of your lifestyle. Sometimes, lifestyle changes alone may not be enough to manage a chronic condition like hypertension. In fact, government statistics indicate that most people require a combination of two medications to get their blood pressure under control. Other chronic conditions like diabetes, high cholesterol levels, and hypertension require a sustained effort to control as well. Diabetics must regulate their blood sugar, or they risk damage to their kidneys and other organs. Cholesterol levels must be controlled to prevent atherosclerosis and dangerous narrowing of the arteries. A healthy adult blood pressure is 120/80 or below; people diagnosed with hypertension need to keep their blood pressure at 140/90 or below. If you have diabetes, your blood pressure should be 130/80 or below. Most importantly, follow the treatment regimen prescribed by your healthcare professional.

Regular medical checkups will also ensure whole-body health and wellness. Risk factors for cardiovascular disease often affect other areas of the body and/or speed the development of other problems like chronic kidney disease or cancer. Early prevention and detection can prolong the quality of your life.

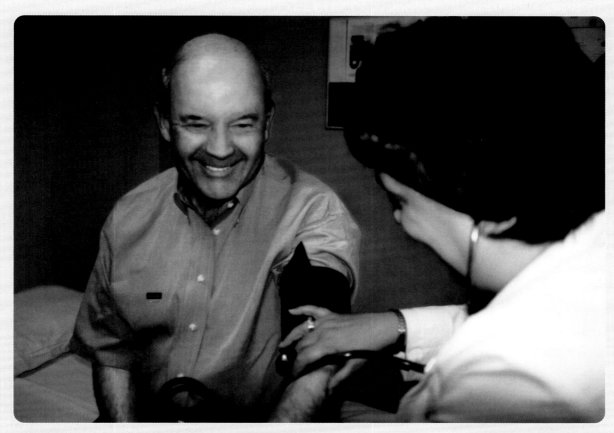

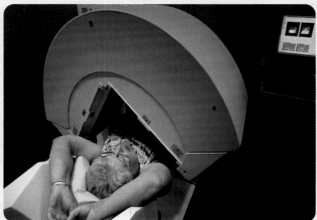

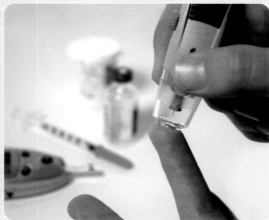

I YEAR OLD

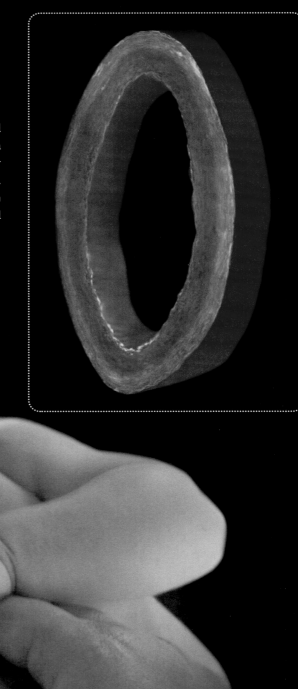

Aging Vessels

It is impossible to avoid the ravages of time. Age-related damage is inevitable, but cardiovascular disease is not a necessary consequence of aging. In many ways, your health and your quality of life are under your control. Chronic conditions such as hypertension and high cholesterol and their consequences can be treated and managed, or better yet, avoided altogether.

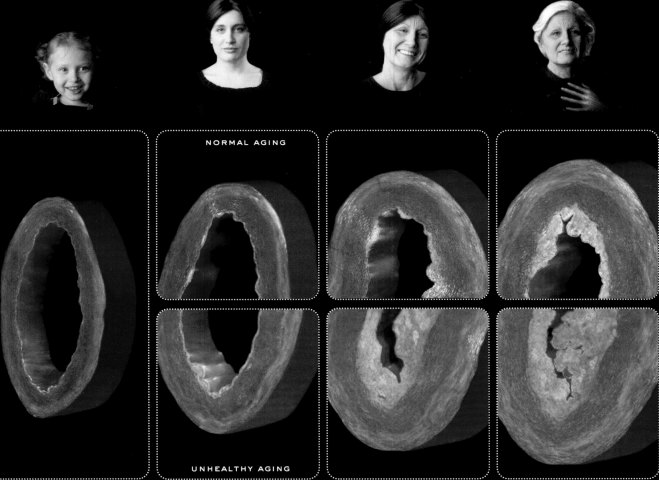

NORMAL AGING

UNHEALTHY AGING

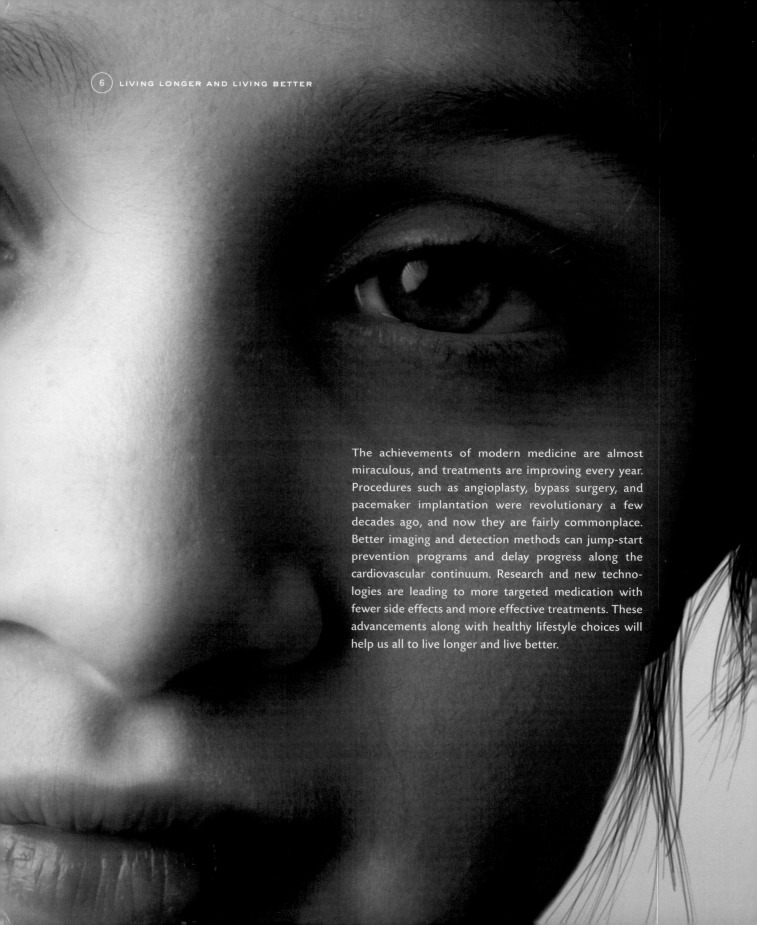

The achievements of modern medicine are almost miraculous, and treatments are improving every year. Procedures such as angioplasty, bypass surgery, and pacemaker implantation were revolutionary a few decades ago, and now they are fairly commonplace. Better imaging and detection methods can jump-start prevention programs and delay progress along the cardiovascular continuum. Research and new technologies are leading to more targeted medication with fewer side effects and more effective treatments. These advancements along with healthy lifestyle choices will help us all to live longer and live better.

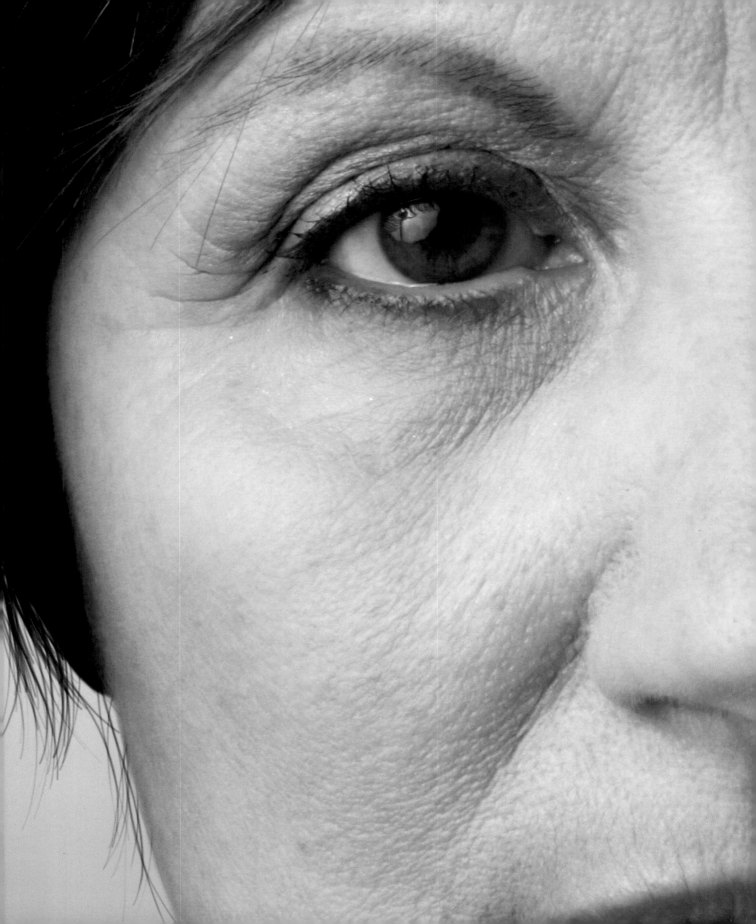

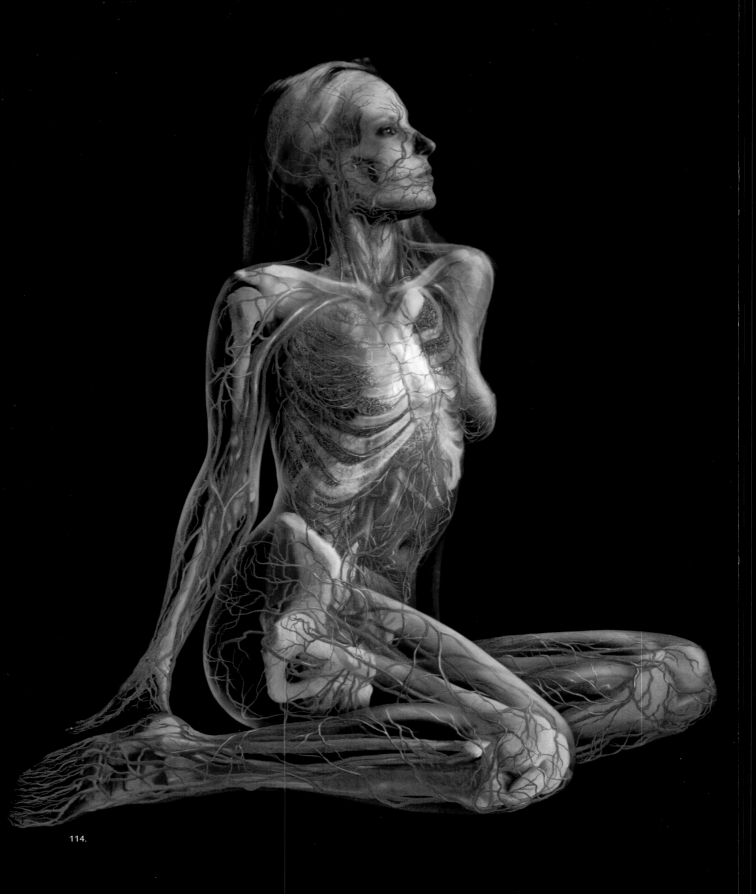

114.

GLOSSARY/INDEX

A

acetylsalicylic acid The active ingredient in aspirin used as a medication to relieve pain and inflammation. 106

adrenaline A hormone released by the body's hormonal glands to prepare for the physical response known as fight or flight. Adrenaline increases heart rate, blood pressure, and blood sugar to provide the body with an energy surge. 89, 104

alveolus, alveoli (pl.) The smallest unit of the lungs; the site of gas exchange with the capillaries. Oxygen and carbon dioxide move between the alveoli to the surrounding capillaries. 36, 37

American Heart Association For more information http://www.americanheart.org. 98, 101

American Society of Hypertension, Inc. For more information http://www.ash-us.org. 45

angina Temporary chest pain or pressure that occurs when the heart muscle is not receiving enough oxygen. 73, 75, 85, 87

angiogram A medical procedure performed to examine blood flow in and around the heart to pinpoint areas of blockage. 75, 76

angioplasty The medical procedure to open blocked arteries. 78, 79, 81, 112

angiotensin A molecule used by the body to control blood vessel contraction and thus blood pressure. 58, 89

angiotensin converting enzyme (ACE) inhibitors Blood pressure lowering medications that decrease the production of angiotensin in the body. 89

angiotensin receptor blockers (ARBs) Blood pressure lowering medications that prohibit the functions of the angiotensin enzyme, which cause blood vessels to contract. These medications also act on the hormones responsible for water balance and sodium regulation. 89

antioxidants Molecules in the body that eliminate free radicals before they can react with and damage cells and DNA. 106

aorta The largest artery in the body leading from the heart. 15, 17

arrhythmia An irregular heartbeat—either too fast (bradycardia) or too slow (tachycardia). Arrhythmia can be caused by heart damage. 57, 85, 87

artery, arteries (pl.) A blood vessel that carries oxygenated blood from the heart to the rest of the body. The exception is the pulmonary artery, which carries deoxygenated blood from the heart to the lungs. 5, 6, 15, 16, 17, 23, 26, 27, 28, 31, 33, 42, 51, 54, 74-81, 86, 87, 95, 109

arteriosclerosis A Greek word that means hardening of the arteries. It can be caused by age, high blood pressure, diabetes, smoking, and high cholesterol levels. 61, 63

atherosclerosis A specific arteriosclerosis condition in which fatty material called plaque develops in the walls of arteries, narrowing the arteries and inhibiting the flow of blood. 64, 69, 70, 71, 72, 75, 86, 87, 90, 95, 97, 98, 99, 109

atrial fibrillation The most common type of arrhythmia or heart rhythm disorder. 57

atrium A chamber of the heart. The right atrium collects deoxygenated blood from the rest of the body and passes it to the right ventricle to be pumped to the lungs. The left atrium collects oxygenated blood from the lungs and passes it to the left ventricle to be pumped to the rest of the body. 12, 17,

atrioventricular (AV) node A specialized bundle of muscle and nerve cells that sits near the bottom of the right atrium. It relays the signal from the sinoatrial (SA) node to the ventricles to contract and pump blood out of the heart. 24, 25

B

baroreceptor A specialized structure of nerve bundles found in arteries that monitors changes in blood pressure and blood flow and provides immediate feedback to the brain. 42, 43

beta blockers Blood pressure lowering medications that work by blocking the effects of adrenaline in the heart. 88, 89

bile acid sequestrants Cholesterol-lowering medications that bind to bile acids and prevent them from being reabsorbed, thus reducing the amount of LDL (bad) cholesterol in the bloodstream. The body needs cholesterol to make bile acids. 90, 91

bladder An organ in the body that stores urine until it is eliminated. 89

blood A complex mixture of plasma, white blood cells, red blood cells and platelets. 4, 5, 9, 11, 12, 151, 6, 17, 19-21, 23, 25, 26, 28, 31, 33-36, 39, 40, 41-43, 45, 47, 48, 54, 56, 57, 63, 70-72, 75, 77, 81, 83, 86, 88-91, 98, 104

blood islands Tiny structures in the yolk sac of embryos that will develop into blood and blood vessels. 9

blood pressure The amount of force the blood exerts on the vessel walls and thus a measure of the health of the cardiovascular system. A blood pressure reading has two numbers. The first (systolic) is the force on the arterial wall generated by the heartbeat. The second number (diastolic) is the force when the heart rests between beats. A healthy adult blood pressure reading is 120/80 or below. 39, 40, 44, 54, 58, 59, 64, 67, 69, 72, 73, 75, 89, 98, 104, 109

blood sugar levels Tightly controlled by the body. Sugar is an energy source; not enough sugar—hypoglycemia—can cause hunger, the shakes, fatigue, and dizziness. Too much sugar—hyperglycemia—is a cardiovascular risk factor that can lead to arteriosclerosis as well as diabetes. 63-65, 67, 69, 104, 109

blood thinner A type of medication that decreases the ability of blood to form clots. 86

body mass index (BMI) A measurement of weight categories based on height. 67

bundle of His Specialized cardiac muscle fibers that transmit signals from the atrioventricular (AV) node to the ventricular muscles of the heart. 24

bypass surgery A surgical procedure that provides a new route for blood flow around areas of blockage in the heart. 80, 81, 112

C

calcium channel blockers Medications that lower blood pressure and relieve angina. They act by selectively blocking the uptake of calcium into the cells. 89

capillary, capillaries (pl.) The smallest blood vessel in the human body. The walls of the capillaries are the primary sites of gas and nutrient exchange. 5, 17, 26, 28, 31-34, 36, 37, 47, 64, 83

cardiovascular continuum The ongoing process of change and remodeling of the cardiovascular system throughout a person's lifetime. 94, 95, 97, 112

catheter A tube used in an angioplasty. The catheter is inserted through an artery in the arm or the groin, and threaded to the area of the blockage. 79

cholesterol A building block for other molecules and components of the body. Cholesterol is made in the liver and obtained from foods. High cholesterol levels increase the risk of atherosclerosis and heart disease. 51, 61, 64, 67, 69, 71, 72, 78, 86, 90-92, 94, 96-99, 101, 109, 110
   LDL (low-density lipoprotein) cholesterol: is often called the bad cholesterol as high levels of LDL cholesterol are linked to such cardiovascular conditions as atherosclerosis and coronary artery disease. 70, 71, 90, 91
   HDL (high-density lipoprotein) cholesterol: is often called the good cholesterol as high levels of HDL cholesterol are believed to protect against coronary artery disease.70, 71, 90, 91, 98

circulation The process by which blood moves through the body.
   pulmonary circulation The right side of the heart—right atrium and right ventricle—sends deoxygenated blood from the heart to the lungs. 15, 19, 20, 36
   systemic circulation The left side of the heart—left atrium and left ventricle—sends oxygenated blood from the heart to the rest of the body. 15, 19, 36

clot A fibrous mass that forms at the sites of injury to stop bleeding. The formation of clots within arteries can slow and block blood flow by decreasing the diameter of the vessel. Clots can also detach and move downstream to block a smaller artery. 51, 75, 79, 86, 87, 98, 104, 106

clot buster A type of medication that dissolves already-formed clots. 86

D

DNA (deoxyribonucleic acid) A double-stranded molecule found primarily in the nuclei of cells. DNA contains the genetic informations and instructions that define the organism. 61, 106

diabetes A health condition in which the body is either unable to produce or to use insulin—a hormone that allows glucose into cells. Glucose is a sugar that is an important energy source in the body. 62-64, 66, 67, 71, 73, 90, 93, 95, 104, 109

dialysis The procedure in which a person is connected to a machine to have his/her blood filtered and cleaned. 54

diastolic (see blood pressure)

diet The foods consumed by a person. 44, 59, 61, 66, 70, 71, 90, 94, 95, 97, 99-101, 106, 107, 109

diuretic A type of drug that enables the kidneys to rid the body of excess fluids. It is often referred to as a water pill. 89

drug compliance The act of taking prescription medication as directed. 93

Ductus arteriosus The opening through which blood can flow from the pulmonary artery directly into the aorta in the fetus. 15-17

E

edema The swelling caused by fluid retention in the body is often a symptom associated with heart failure. 83
   pedel edema Swelling of the legs.
   pulmonary edema A condition where fluid collects in the lungs and can interfere with breathing.

electrocardiogram (ECG) A test that measures the electrical impulses flowing through the heart. 24, 25, 56, 57, 74, 85

embryo An organism in an early stage of development

endothelial cell A cell type used as lining in many parts of the body. Endothelial cells line the inside of blood vessels. 31, 72

erythrocyte (see red blood cell)

exercise Any physical activity that elevates the heart rate for a sustained period of time. 19, 60, 63, 67, 70, 85, 94, 95, 100, 101, 105, 109

F

fatty streak The early sign of atherosclerosis seen in the lining of arteries. 72

fetus In humans, a developing organism from eight weeks after conception until birth. 8-10, 14-16

fibrate A type of medication that can increase the level of HDL cholesterol, which then lowers LDL levels. Fibrates also increase the breakdown of triglycerides. 90, 91

folic acid A compound that controls the levels of homocysteine in the blood. Green leafy vegetables are high in folic acid. 98

Foramen ovale The opening in the fetus that allows blood to flow from the right side of the heart directly into the left side of the heart. 15-17

Framingham Heart Study The groundbreaking study involving subjects from the town of Framingham in Massachusetts. The study has uncovered many of the known cardiovascular risk factors. 61, 63, 67, 69, 94

free radicals Atoms or a group of atoms with unpaired electrons. They can be formed when oxygen interacts with certain molecules and also through exposure to pollution, radiation, or cigarette smoke. Free radicals can damage cells and DNA. 106, 107

G

glomerulus, glomeruli (pl.) A specialized structure in the kidney made up of capillaries. Blood is filtered through the glomeruli. 34, 35

H

heart attack (a.k.a. myocardial infarction) A condition when blood flow to the heart is reduced or blocked. Heart cells die when the blood supply is cut off; the longer the blood supply is cut off, the greater the area of heart damage. 45, 61, 64, 73, 75, 78, 81, 82, 85, 86, 95, 98, 102, 105, 106, 109

heart failure A condition in which the ventricles of the heart are unable to pump blood effectively. 81, 83, 85

heart rate The number of times the heart beats per minute. 19, 42

heart tube The structure in embryos that will eventually develop into a four-chambered human heart. 12, 13

hemoglobin The iron-containing protein in red blood cells that binds oxygen and carbon dioxide for transport and delivery to different parts of the body. 36, 37

high blood pressure (see hypertension)

homocysteine An amino acid that can cause nicks in the arterial wall, and thus promote the development of atherosclerosis. 98

hypertension (a.k.a. high blood pressure) One of the main indicators (and causes) of cardiovascular disease. A healthy adult blood pressure reading is 120/80 mm Hg. For every increase of 20 in the first number or 10 in the second, the cardiovascular risk doubles. 38-40, 45-49, 54-59, 61, 62, 66, 67, 70, 71, 78, 89, 90, 92, 93, 95, 97, 100, 109, 110

I

insulin A hormone produced by the pancreas used to control blood sugar levels. 63, 69

ischemia An inadequate supply of blood to an area of the body. 51, 95

K

kidney The organ that filters wastes from the blood. 6, 19, 34, 54, 55, 58, 62-64, 67, 88, 89, 93, 95, 109

L

left ventricular hypertrophy The condition in which the left ventricle becomes thickened and enlarged, often resulting from severe and prolonged hypertension. 56

Lehigh Valley Hospital and Health Network For more information http://www.lvhhn.org. 86, 92, 95

lipoprotein (see cholesterol)

Lowering of Vascular Atherosclerotic Risk (LOVAR) 95, 99, 101, 109

M

mitochondria Cellular organelles that provides energy to the cell. 31

N

nephron A functional unit of the kidney. 35

New York Presbyterian-Columbia University Hospital For more information http://www.nyp.org/. 2, 21

niacin A type of cholesterol-lowering medication. Niacins increase the level of HDL cholesterol, which then lowers LDL levels. 90, 91

nicotine The active ingredient in cigarette smoke. Nicotine increases blood pressure and can block the release of insulin, thus increasing blood sugar levels. 60, 69

nitroglycerin A medication often prescribed for angina. Nitroglycerin works quickly to dilate the blood vessels and increase blood flow to the heart. 83

noradrenaline A chemical messenger that increases heart rate. 89

O

obese/obesity A condition in which the individual is 30 or more pounds heavier than recommended for their height. Refer to body mass index (BMI). 66, 67, 94

omega-3 fatty acid A type of polyunsaturated fatty acid, which has been shown to make blood less likely to clot, thus lowering the risk of heart attacks and strokes. Omega-3 fatty acids also lower blood pressure and triglyceride levels, and increase good HDL cholesterol levels. 98

osteoporosis The condition where bone mass is lost, making bones more brittle and prone to breakage. 105

oxidative stress The damage caused by free radicals. 106

P

pacemaker A device that can be surgically implanted in the chest to help regulate heart beat. 84, 85, 112

pancreas An organ near the stomach that secretes digestive fluids into the intestine and produces the hormone insulin. 62, 63

pericyte A contractile cell scattered throughout the capillary walls. 31

placenta The organ consisting of the umbilical cord and surrounding tissues that links the mother and the growing fetus during pregnancy. The placenta provides nutrients to the fetus and takes away wastes. 9, 10, 15

plaque A deposit of fats, inflammatory cells, proteins, and calcium material along the inner lining of arteries. The buildup of these deposits can narrow the diameter of arteries, thus slowing and/or blocking blood flow and raising blood pressure. 51-53, 69, 70, 72, 75, 78, 79, 86, 87, 90

R

red blood cells (a.k.a. erythrocytes) The primary oxygen transporters. Mature red blood cells are the only cells in the body with no nuclei. 33, 36

retina The tissue at the back of the eye that transmits visual images through the optic nerve to the brain. 46, 47

S

saturated fats Fats that are often solid at room temperature. Most animal fats are saturated and can increase blood cholesterol levels. 96, 97, 98

sinoatrial (SA) node A specialized bundle of muscle and nerve cells that sits at the top of the right atrium. It is the pacemaker of the heart and generates the signal for the atria to contract and send blood to the ventricles. 24, 25

statin A type of cholesterol-lowering medication, which inhibits the production of the enzyme that makes cholesterol. 78, 90 91, 106

stent A wire-mesh netting that can be left in place during an angioplasty to keep the artery open. 27, 76, 78, 79, 104

stress management Strategies used to handle the pressures of life. 104, 108

stroke A condition in which there is a disruption of blood flow to the brain either because of a blockage or a ruptured artery. With the loss of blood supply, brain cells die and areas of the brain are damaged. 39, 40, 48

    embolic stroke The instance when a clot breaks off from its original site and moves through the bloodstream to block one of the smaller arteries in the brain. 86

    hemorrhagic stroke The instance when a blood vessel in the brain ruptures. 50, 51

    ischemic stroke The instance when blockage occurs in the arteries leading to, and within, the brain either due to a clot or narrowing of the arteries from advanced atherosclerosis. 51

    thrombotic stroke The instance when a clot forms in the artery and blocks blood flow to the brain. 86

    transient ischemic attacks (TIAs) Mini-strokes that occur when the blood supply to an area of the brain is cut off, or vastly decreased, for a short period of time. 86

sudden cardiac death A sudden, unexpected death caused by loss of heart function. 84

systolic pressure (see Blood pressure)

T

transient ischemic attack (TIA) (see stroke)

triglyceride A type of fat found in the blood. Most fat found in the diet and body is in the form of triglycerides. 90, 97, 98

Tunica adventitia: The outermost layer of cells that makes up an artery or a vein. 31

Tunica intima The innermost layer of cells that makes up an artery or vein. 31

Tunica media The middle layer of cells that makes up an artery or vein. 31

U

UCLA Center for Cholesterol and Lipid Management For more information http://www.healthcare.ucla.edu/institution/groups-detail?group_id=13061. 54

umbilical cord The structure that together with other tissues makes up the placenta, and is the link between the mother and the developing fetus during pregnancy. 9, 10, 15

United States Department of Agriculture (USDA) For more information http://www.usda.gov. 98, 101

V

valve A structure that maintains the direction of blood flow. 15, 20, 22, 23, 31, 111

Vascular Improvement Plan for Life® (VIP) For more information http://www.lvh.org/vipforlife/. 95, 99, 109

vein A blood vessel that carries deoxygenated blood to the heart from the rest of the body. The exception is the pulmonary vein, which carries oxygenated blood from the lungs to the heart. 5, 17, 27, 28, 31, 77, 80, 81, 83

ventricle A chamber of the heart. The right ventricle pumps deoxygenated blood to the lungs. The left ventricle pumps oxygenated blood from the lungs to the rest of the body. 12, 17, 20, 23, 25, 41, 56

vitamin An organic compound usually derived from food that is essential for metabolism. There are different types of vitamins used by the body for different purposes. 106

Y

yoga A type of exercise of Hindu origin that practices control of the mind and body. 105

yolk sac A food source for the early embryo during development. 9

INTRODUCING THE INVISION GUIDE SERIES, THE DRAMATIC NEW WAY TO LOOK AT YOUR HEALTH

This book offers a fabulous, full-color journey through the cardiovascular system using a groundbreaking visual technology that sees into body tissue in many dimensions and at multiple points in time. The result: stunning visuals that are not merely reflections of the surface (of a blood cell, artery, or a heart valve), but are dimensional renderings.

In this visually driven health book, we see:
- the development of the cardiovascular system from conception to birth,
- the marvel of the adult cardiovascular system and how it works,
- how hypertension and other risk factors insidiously damage this beautiful, powerful system, and
- surgical, medical, and lifestyle strategies for cardiovascular health.

By showing the astonishing beauty of the heart in action, this inspiring book makes the urgency of maintaining heart health real and relevant as never before.

The marvels of the human anatomy and the alterations that occur with increased blood pressure are demonstrated in a grand fashion in this wonderful depiction of the cardiovascular system. This atlas will serve as an admirable bridge for communication to all those involved in the treatment of hypertension, from patients to medical personnel. The artwork is superb and easy to grasp and the text provides easy-to-read clarifying detail. A must for those involved in the management of hypertension and cardiovascular disease."

—THOMAS GILES, M.D., *President, American Society of Hypertension, Inc. (ASH)*

Nurses are committed to helping their patients learn new strategies to improve their health and well being. The visual content of this patient-focused book will assist nurses in educating their patients to learn about the serious effects of high blood pressure and cardiovascular disease."

—BARBARA A. BLAKENEY, M.S., R.N., *President, American Nurses Association (ANA)*

This is awesome! I am glad I live at a time when it is possible to see images like this. These amazing images will be the talk of the town for their natural beauty and will help to educate physicians and other scholars, students, patients, and just about anyone who is amazed by the beauty and accurate depictions and illustrations of the human body. Congratulations; this is truly wonderful."

—B. WAINE KONG, PH.D., J.D., *Chief Executive Officer, Association of Black Cardiologists, Inc. (ABC)*

ALEXANDER TSIARAS, FOUNDER/CEO, ANATOMICAL TRAVELOGUE, INC.
Alexander Tsiaras, founder and CEO of Anatomical Travelogue, Inc., has more than twenty years of experience in the worlds of medicine, research, and art, and has won world recognition as a photojournalist, artist, and writer. His work has been featured on numerous television programs and on the covers of *Life, Time, The New York Times Magazine, Smithsonian*, and many other magazines. He is the author of *From Conception to Birth: A Life Unfolds*, and *The Architecture and Design of Man and Woman: The Marvel of the Human Body, Revealed.* Mr. Tsiaras lives in Ne

MEDICAL/Cardiology

ISBN-13: 978-0-06-085593-2
ISBN-10: 0-06-085593-2

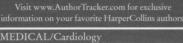
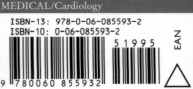

51995

9 780060 855932

EAN

USA $19.95/Canada $26.95

0905

Collins
An Imprint of HarperCollinsPublishers
www.harpercollins.com

Visit the companion website:
http://www.invisionguide.com/heart